Praise for *Drugs - without the hot air*

- *"The most sensible book about drugs you'll read this year ... Nutt is both committed to rigorous, evidence-based policy and to clear, no-nonsense prose that makes complex subjects comprehensible... a book that everyone should read."*
  Cory Doctorow, BoingBoing

- *"This hugely accessible book should be compulsory reading for all who have concerns about the use of recreational drugs ... I cannot praise this book enough."*
  The Pharmaceutical Journal

- *"Finally, Drug Education Gets Real ... There's an inherent danger in any sector of education: if the teachings fail to measure up to the truth, then we'll be paving the way for a deep distrust and a greater apathy. With this in mind, it is of tremendous enthusiasm that we welcome Professor Nutt's book: Drugs - Without the Hot Air "*
  Huffington Post

- *"Bans on drugs like ecstasy, magic mushrooms and LSD have hampered scientific research on the brain and stalled the progress of medicine as much as George Bush's ban on stem cell research did, a leading British drug expert said"*
  Reuters, London

- *"David Nutt is one of those rare scientists with equal talent for making the complex accessible and for telling a great story. The result is so much more than a wonderful cornucopia of information and evidence about drugs, its also a thoroughly engaging read. "*
  Public Health Today

Drugs – without the hot air

Minimising the harms
of legal and illegal drugs

David Nutt

UIT

CAMBRIDGE, ENGLAND

Published by
UIT Cambridge Ltd.
PO Box 145
Cambridge
CB4 1GQ
England

Tel: +44 1223 302 041
Web: www.uit.co.uk

ISBN 9781906860165 (paperback)
ISBN 9781906860400, 9781906860509, 9781906860608 (ebooks)

Contents at a glance

Contents

Preface

Chapter endnotes

To avoid interrupting the flow of reading, the book contains no footnotes. Instead, there are detailed lists of sources and references at the end of each chapter. In the text, a mark (†) indicates the *start* of the text that the note relates to, and the chapter's endnote repeats the page number and the original text, followed by the text of the note. For example, on page 1, "†a lecture I'd given a few months before", points to the note "1 a lecture I'd given a few months before • *Estimating Drug Harms: A Risky Business?*, David Nutt, URL-2, October 10th 2009", which appears at the end of the chapter, on page 7.

When reading the book for the first time, you may not want to bother with the endnotes as they often refer to specialist publications or articles. However, you will find them useful when you want to verify something in the text, or to find more information on a topic.

URLs and web links

To save space and duplication, URLs for webpages are shown like this: URL-2, with the full text of the corresponding web link given in the list of URLs on page 317.

Acknowledgement

The author and publisher give special thanks to Deborah Grayson for her tireless work as project editor for this book.

1 Why I had to write this book

†**Tom Brake MP**: *Does the Prime Minister believe that once a healthier relationship is established between politicians and the media, it will be easier for Governments to adopt evidence-based policy in relation to, for instance, tackling drugs?*

David Cameron: *That is a lovely idea.*

Many people who don't recognise my name or know anything about my work will nonetheless remember me as "the scientist who got sacked". In many ways my departure from the government's Advisory Council on the Misuse of Drugs is where this book began, so it makes sense to start the story there.

In October 2009, †a lecture I'd given a few months before was released as a pamphlet on the internet. For some reason – perhaps it was a slow news day – this got picked up by the media and I was invited on to BBC Radio 4 for an interview. This generated more interest and several more interviews. A few days later I got an e-mail from the then Home Secretary Alan Johnson asking me to resign from my position as chair of the Advisory Council on the Misuse of Drugs (ACMD). When I refused he released a statement saying that I had been sacked.

The lecture that sparked off this chain of events had covered a number of topics, but all the media wanted to talk about were my views on cannabis. In January 2009, against the recommendation of the ACMD, after four years in Class C, cannabis was re-upgraded to Class B, indicating increased harmfulness. Jacqui Smith, who was Home Secretary at the time, justified ignoring the recommendations of our report because, she said, her †*"decision takes into account issues such as public perception and the needs and consequences for policing priorities. ... Where there is ... doubt about the potential harm that will be caused, we must err on the side of caution and*

1

protect the public." In the lecture, I discussed whether this was a rational approach, and particularly whether putting a drug in a higher legal Class in order to "err on the side of caution" would actually protect the public and reduce harm.

I'd called the lecture *Estimating Drug Harms: a Risky Business?* because I knew from experience that talking about the harm done by drugs in relative terms was considered politically sensitive. This had been made very clear to me when a scientific editorial I'd written the year before, comparing the harms of ecstasy with those of horse riding, provoked questions in Parliament and an unhappy personal call from Jacqui. (You can read more about this episode on page 20.)

There had been a similar reaction to a [†]paper I co-wrote in 2007, which tried to rank 20 drugs in order of harmfulness, taking into account 9 different sorts of harm, including physical, psychological and social factors. Politicians didn't like the idea of some drugs being openly acknowledged as "less harmful" than others (or even worse, less harmful than legal drugs such as alcohol), in case it encouraged more people to use them, or made the politicians seem less "tough" in the eyes of the tabloids. This is despite the fact that the *point* of having different Classes of drugs built into the Misuse of Drugs Act was to communicate to the public a degree of relative harm [†](Table 1.1). Class B drugs should be less harmful than Class As, and Class C drugs less harmful than Class Bs. Incidentally, many drugs that have medical uses are both covered by the Misuse of Drugs Act, and regulated by the Medicines and Healthcare products Regulatory Agency (MHRA) and the Medicines Act (Figure 1.1).

Class	Includes	Possession	Dealing
A	Ecstasy, LSD, heroin, cocaine, crack, magic mushrooms, amphetamines (injected)	7 years	Life
B	Amphetamines, cannabis, Ritalin	5 years	14 years
C	Tranquillisers, some painkillers, GHB, ketamine	2 years	14 years

Table 1.1: The maximum prison sentences laid down by the Misuse of Drugs Act.

Which brings us back to cannabis – the only drug in the history of the Misuse of Drugs Act ever to be downgraded, following recommenda-

Drugs – without the hot air, David Nutt

tions made by the [†]Runciman report in the year 2000. After the down-grading of cannabis, however, the media, along with some politicians and medical professionals, became concerned that stronger forms of the drug (known as "skunk") were causing serious mental illnesses such as schizophrenia.

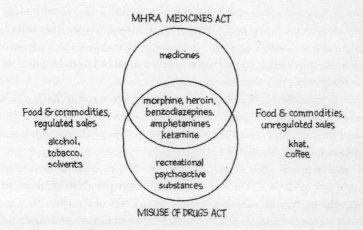

Figure 1.1: Many drugs are controlled as both medicines and as illegal drugs.

There was certainly a legitimate question as to whether new breeds of cannabis were more harmful than the sort that had been considered by Runciman and the ACMD in the past. As the government's advisory council, this is exactly the sort of issue that our research was supposed to address, and we undertook a very thorough study – one of the most comprehensive ever. Our conclusion was that, although there probably was a causal link between smoking cannabis and some cases of schizophrenia, this link was weak and didn't justify moving the drug up to the next Class. Yes, there was a risk of developing a serious mental illness after using the drug, but it was smaller than the risks posed by other Class Bs such as amphetamines, which can also cause psychosis. This was the message that we wanted to send to the public by keeping cannabis in Class C.

Certainly, nobody was calling cannabis safe. However, as my 2007 report had shown, across a range of different sorts of harm it was by no means as damaging as many other drugs, particularly alcohol. This was a point I made in my lecture, and which got picked up in the radio interview: *"surely you can't be saying alcohol is more harmful than cannabis?"* I replied yes, that's exactly what I'm saying, it's there in my 2007 paper, which at the time was reported on the front page of the *Independent* and the *Guardian* so it was hardly a secret. But this question was repeated in the other interviews that week – everybody wanted the quote that alcohol was more harmful than cannabis. It seemed like an entirely defensible thing to say, as it was based on my own scientific work, and backed up by a similar study from Holland which had agreed that alcohol deserved to be ranked among the most harmful of drugs. In these interviews I also observed that the government had asked the ACMD to determine which Class cannabis belonged in, and then hadn't followed our advice.

†In a letter to the *Guardian* a few days after he sacked me, Alan Johnson explained that I *"was asked to go because he cannot be both a government adviser and a campaigner against government policy."* †I responded in *The Times* that I didn't understand what he meant when he said I had crossed the line from science to policy, and that I did not know where this line was. The ACMD was *supposed* to advise on policy, and indeed it was set up by the Misuse of Drugs Act because even in the 1970s it was known that politicians liked to play party politics with drugs regulation. Of course, politicians have to take into account issues beyond "pure" scientific evidence in many of their decisions, but the legal Class of a drug is supposed to inform the public about relative harm, and those who designed the Act recognised this was best determined by a group of independent experts. By acting against our recommendations, the Brown government had themselves blurred the line between science and policy.

The subtitle of this book refers to minimising the harm done by drugs. This has always been my primary concern as a psychiatrist, and what I always hoped the ACMD was working towards. The upgrading of cannabis to Class B was the third time we had been ignored. (The other two were when magic mushrooms were made Class A without consulting

Drugs – without the hot air, David Nutt

us, and when the government refused to downgrade ecstasy to Class B despite our recommendation.) The longer the government went on creating policies that conflicted with the scientific evidence, the more harm those policies would do, not least because they undermined our ability to give a consistent public-health message, especially around the dangers of alcohol. The more hysterical and exaggerated any Home Secretary was about the harms of cannabis, the less credibility they would have in the eyes of the teenagers binge-drinking themselves into comas every day. If we're going to minimise harm, we have to have a way of measuring it, and a policy framework that can respond to this evidence. Yet even comparing the dangers of cannabis and alcohol was considered a "political" act that overstepped my remit as a scientist and physician.

I am not the only scientist to have suffered the displeasure of the Brown government. A couple of years ago, the Chief Medical Officer (CMO) Sir Liam Donaldson warned of the rapidly-growing medical costs of alcohol use and recommended [†]a sensible policy of increasing the price of the cheapest drinks. His report was dismissed in an insulting manner by the Labour government, leading to his leaving the post of CMO early. The past-president of the Royal College of Physicians [†]Sir Ian Gilmore was also ridiculed by much of the press and parts of government when he shared his view that the current drug laws were not working, and that the personal use of drugs should be decriminalised as in Portugal.

The day after I was sacked, I received an email from Toby Jackson, a man with a keen interest in science, who was in the fortunate position of being rather wealthy. He was horrified by my treatment and offered to fund an alternative to the ACMD that could carry out drugs research free from political interference. Together, we founded the Independent Scientific Committee on Drugs (ISCD), and most of the scientific experts who resigned from the ACMD as a result of my sacking have joined us on the team. (A few members have also worked with both councils simultaneously.) Being outside government has in many ways been a blessing, as it has allowed us to be far more outspoken in our criticism of government policies, notably during the mephedrone debacle. My hope is that this book can put some of the ISCD's work in context, and help contribute to a debate about drugs – including alcohol and tobacco – which is grounded in objective evidence.

Who this book is for

This book is framed around controversial issues such as the banning of mephedrone, whether alcohol is more harmful than many illegal drugs, and whether addiction can be cured. Along the way, we'll learn how different drugs work, why we take them and what the future might hold. The focus is largely on what are usually considered "recreational" drugs, but almost all have medical uses as well, and there is a chapter on therapeutics like antidepressants. My primary aim is to help you become better informed about the harms of taking drugs, as well as the benefits, so that you can make better decisions about the risks you want to take with your own body (and perhaps with your career and family life). Even if you're not the sort of person who'd consider taking illegal drugs, you'll still need to make decisions about alcohol, coffee, tobacco, and medication prescribed by your doctor. There's a chapter at the end aimed at parents, to help them talk to their children about drugs, but I hope a lot of the "kids" themselves will be reading this, too.

You don't need any specialist knowledge to understand this book: it doesn't assume you have any prior experience in medical or drugs matters. At the back of the book there are suggestions for further reading if you want to look into any of the topics in more detail. There is also a full list of the webpages we reference; this list is also on the book's website (uit.co.uk/drugs) to make it easy to access the references online.

While everything in this book is grounded in scientific evidence, drugs also have social and cultural aspects. We can't talk about reducing the harms drugs cause without examining how they are used, how freely available they are, and their legal status. So this is also a book about policies – the ones that reduce harms (like the smoking ban), and the ones that increase them (like allowing cut-price alcohol in supermarkets). Inevitably, the book is critical of the "War on Drugs" (chapter 15), not just because this set of policies has caused enormous damage to millions of people around the world, but also because the evidence of the harm it has been causing hasn't led to a change of approach. Politicians must often make decisions with imperfect knowledge, and sometimes those decisions don't work or have unintended negative consequences. The War on Drugs wasn't so obviously the wrong thing to try in the 1970s, but today it is clearly doing more harm than good, and the "drugs problem" needs radical rethinking as a public-health crisis rather than a moral crusade.

When I first started working with the government, I thought that our drugs policies were broadly going in the right direction. As time went by and I realised the extent of the perverse consequences the policies were causing, I came to the conclusion that the Misuse of Drugs Act is no longer fit for purpose and needed to be thoroughly revised. The crucial point is that *I changed my mind*. Being willing to change our minds in the light of new evidence is essential to rational policy-making. As long as our politicians refuse to consider any framework other than prohibition and criminalisation, then science and evidence will be considered dangerous, and those who champion them will be sidelined and even sacked. I hope that this book will contribute to a new understanding of the issues around drugs that is rational, scientific and humane.

Notes

Page

1 **Tom Brake MP**: *Does the Prime Minister believe* •Phone Hacking Oral Answers to Questions – Prime Minister, Tom Brake MP, URL-1, July 13th 2011. Follow the link at URL-1 to see Tom Brake's question in context.

1 a lecture I'd given a few months before• *Estimating Drug Harms: A Risky Business?*, David Nutt, URL-2, October 10th 2009

1 *"decision takes into account issues such as public perception and the needs and consequences for policing priorities.*•URL-2 as above.

2 paper I co-wrote in 2007• *Development of a rational scale to assess the harm of drugs of potential misuse*, Nutt et al, Lancet, 2007

2 (Table 1.1)• *Class A, B and C drugs*, Home Office, URL-177.

3 Runciman report• *Drugs and the law*, Report of the Independent Inquiry into the Misuse of Drugs Act, Chairman Viscountess Runciman, URL-3, 2000

4 In a letter to the *Guardian*• *Why Prof David Nutt was shown the door*, Alan Johnson, URL-4, November 2nd 2009

4 I responded in *The Times*• *Penalties for drug use must reflect harm*, David Nutt, URL-5, November 2, 2009

5 a sensible policy of increasing the price of the cheapest drinks• *Chief Medical Officer vows to press on with anti-alcohol campaign, despite No. 10 rebuff*, Sam Lister, URL-6, March 17th 2009

5 Sir Ian Gilmore was also ridiculed by much of the press and parts of government• *Top doctor Sir Ian Gilmore calls for drugs law review*, BBC news, URL-7, August 17th 2010

2 Is ecstasy more dangerous than horse riding?

The field I work in is called psychopharmacology – I specialise in using drugs to help people with brain problems. A few years ago, I began treating a middle-aged woman who came to see me with brain damage. Her personality had changed after a head injury, and she was now irritable, anxious, and occasionally aggressive. Her impulsive and difficult behaviour had led to her children being taken into care, and she was banned from her local pub after abusing the staff and customers. She'd left her job, and was unlikely to be able to work ever again. The brain damage had seriously and permanently affected her life, and had imposed some very high costs on society.

Part of my clinical work is with people suffering from addictions to drugs, and her story would be familiar to many people dependent on drugs or other substances, but this woman's neurological damage had been caused by something else entirely: a bad fall from a horse. I treated the patient with a type of amphetamine that helped manage some of the symptoms, but I was interested to find that an activity as apparently wholesome as horse riding could be so dangerous. I started to look into the statistics, and found them quite startling.

Every year in the UK around [†]10 people die while horse riding, and there are over [†]100 road traffic accidents involving horses which often result in deaths as well. Falls onto the neck and spine can lead to permanent spinal injuries, and head injuries can lead to irreversible brain damage, as my patient experienced. In some shire counties where the sport is very common, it is well-recognised as a leading cause of early-onset Parkinson's disease. Studies in the USA have calculated there are approximately 11,500 cases of traumatic head injury each year due to riding.

In the UK, [†]research from the National Spinal Injuries Centre at Stoke Mandeville hospital shows a rider can expect a serious accident once in every 350 hours riding. If we assume that there are [†]2 million riding episodes a year, that gives us about 5,700 serious accidents. And although more experienced riders are probably more aware of the dangers, they are also more likely to take risks and suffer injuries and take part in the most dangerous forms of cross-country racing. (Eventing and fox-hunting are more risky than other sorts of riding, because of the jumps.)

Go compare

Looking at these figures, I began to suspect that horse riding might be considerably more harmful than some drugs that are currently illegal. I decided to see whether I could compare the dangers of getting on a horse, with the dangers of taking ecstasy – a Class A drug popular with club-goers. If the probability of something bad happening was 1 in 350 for horse riding, what was the equivalent probability for taking an ecstasy pill? I'd need to find comparable data for the adverse events on horse-back: deaths, injuries, road traffic accidents. I would also need to take into account some of the special features of drugs, such as the risk of addiction, and factor-in social problems such as violent behaviour. Even if I couldn't find precise numbers, I thought I could get a rough idea of the scale of the harm caused by each activity, in order to try and work out which was more dangerous.

I began by estimating the number of people ecstasy kills each year. The numbers vary slightly depending on where you get your figures from, but coroners' reports list [†]ecstasy as the sole cause of death for 10–17 people a year, and it's mentioned on the death certificates of 33–50 others. Most people who take ecstasy are "poly drug users" (meaning they take other things at the same time), and just because they had ecstasy in their system when they died doesn't mean it necessarily contributed to their deaths. So I took a rough estimate of 10–50 deaths a year.

I then looked for data on ecstasy and road traffic accidents. There didn't seem to be much information on this, perhaps because the police

Drugs – without the hot air, David Nutt

don't test for it very regularly, but I did find some laboratory studies where people simulated driving while under the influence of ecstasy alone, and after taking ecstasy and alcohol together. These showed that although the drug impairs some aspects of driving performance, it actually improves things like attention and concentration, and this was particularly marked when combined with alcohol. Given the lack of clear data either way, I decided to omit ecstasy-related traffic accidents.

To compare with the number of head injuries from horse riding, I looked back at the report on ecstasy we produced in 2008 when I was still chair of the ACMD, where we estimated that the drug was in some way involved in a couple of thousand hospital admissions every year. Most of these were pretty mild, or primarily caused by co-ingestants (ie other drugs taken at the same time, such as alcohol or GHB), but a few each year were serious, ecstasy-specific, injuries such as liver damage. I picked a rough figure of [†]2,000 serious but non-fatal injuries from ecstasy every year, which was likely to be an overestimate.

Of course, becoming addicted is one of the biggest dangers posed by drugs, and while ecstasy doesn't cause a physical withdrawal syndrome, psychological dependence isn't unknown. About [†]1,000 of those who seek specialist treatment for drug dependence every year say it's the main drug they're abusing, which probably represents about half of those addicted to ecstasy, as not everybody seeks professional help. (Although not strictly an addiction, the pleasure of riding is so great that many people want to continue the sport even after causing themselves harm. [†]Melanie Reid, the *Times* journalist who broke her neck falling from a horse in 2010, has described her longing to ride again in terms very reminiscent of drug use.)

Another big concern is that people under the influence of drugs might behave antisocially. However, aggression is very rare in ecstasy users, and if any do become violent it's almost certainly because of other drugs they've taken (such as alcohol). This indirect association is similar to the relationship between horse riding and the occasional violence when hunters clash with hunt saboteurs. Antisocial behaviour doesn't seem to be a significant source of harm for either activity.

Different sorts of harm	Ecstasy (60 m episodes/yr)	Horse riding (2 m episodes/yr)
Deaths	10–50 deaths/yr	10 deaths/yr, plus some fatal road traffic accidents
Physical damage	2,000 hospital admissions	100 non-fatal road traffic accidents, 5,700 serious accidents
Addictiveness	1,000 seek treatment every year, 1,000 others are also addicted	Not really applicable
Psychological damage	Ecstasy can cause mild cognitive impairment for heavy users, memory problems, occasionally people have visual hallucinations and panic attacks. There's a weak link to depression	Memory loss, personality change, early onset Parkinson's disease
Loss of tangibles and relationships	Rare cases	Rare cases like my patient
Injury to others	Very little	Road traffic accidents, occasional aggression between hunters and hunt saboteurs
Crime	Not much, apart from dealing and supply of drug itself	Illegal hunts
Economic cost	Treating injuries on the NHS	Treating injuries on the NHS
Total	**About 6,000/yr**	**About 6,000/yr**

Table 2.1: A comparison of the harms of ecstasy and horse riding.

The total number of "adverse events" for ecstasy and horse riding were very similar in the end – perhaps about 6,000 cases every year (Table 2.1). Ecstasy pills, however, are far more common than riding, with police estimating that about [†]60 million tablets are taken every year. 6,000 out of 60 million means that ecstasy causes roughly one case of [†]acute harm every 10,000 episodes: every 10,000th pill, someone is likely to get hurt. This is obviously a very rough estimate, but was so much *less* likely than getting hurt every 350 episodes that I felt confident saying that horse riding was a more dangerous activity.

Drugs – without the hot air, David Nutt

Equasy

In 2009, I wrote an [†]editorial in the *Journal of Psychopharmacology* comparing the harms caused by ecstasy to those of a made-up affliction called "equasy", short for "equine addiction syndrome". I pointed out how dangerous equasy was, and suggested that we consider banning horse riding as a harm-reduction measure – adding that this would be far more practical than banning drugs as it's hard to ride a horse in the privacy of your own home! Apart from a few readers of the *Horse and Hound*, most people understood that this was tongue in cheek: I was making a point that criminalising risky behaviour is only one way to reduce harm, and not always the most appropriate way. The comparison with ecstasy was also intended to highlight the fact that the drug debate takes place without reference to other causes of harm in society, which tends to give drugs a different, more subjectively-worrying, status.

As chair of the Advisory Council on the Misuse of Drugs at the time, I suppose I knew that this would provoke a response from government, but I didn't expect a personal call from the then Home Secretary, Jacqui Smith, asking me to apologise, or for my editorial to be mentioned in the House of Commons. In a speech shortly after publication, she said that my piece [†]*"makes light of a serious problem, trivialises the dangers of drugs, shows insensitivity to the families of victims of ecstasy and sends the wrong message to young people about the dangers of drugs."* A Conservative MP joined in, saying that drug use and horse riding were [†]*"completely incomparable"*, and that I was in the *"wrong job"*.

This seemed like something of an overreaction. After all, I had only compared two sets of figures already freely available, and suggested that they might help us to think in a different way about our approach to drugs. I certainly didn't mean to trivialise the pain experienced by those who had lost family members to ecstasy, and did make a public apology to that effect – although I maintain that the suffering of my patient and her family as a result of her horse riding accident was also very severe. But the fact that two thousand words in a scientific journal could provoke so much hostility seemed to speak volumes about our approach to the subject of drug harms. To understand why people objected so strongly to the suggestion that taking ecstasy might be a rational choice, comparable to the rational choice of taking part in a risky sport such as horse riding, we need to look at the history of the drug, learn more about its effects, and understand its particular place in the media.

What is ecstasy?

Ecstasy is the colloquial name for the chemical compound 3,4-methylene-dioxymethylamphetamine (MDMA) which is commonly sold as a pill or powder. It was first synthesised in Germany in 1912 as a weight-loss drug, but was largely ignored until the 1960s when it began to be used as an aid to psychotherapy. Its chemical structure is similar to both amphetamines and some psychedelics, and it was made illegal in the UK in 1977 because of a supposed similarity to LSD (although in fact ecstasy very rarely produces hallucinations). In the 1960s, the drug was known as "empathy", and it didn't seem to occur to anyone to use it recreationally. It was only in the 1980s, when someone had the brainwave of re-branding it "ecstasy" and started to sell it at dance clubs, that it came into popular use. Like amphetamines, ecstasy gave users huge amounts of energy so they could keep dancing all night. But like psychedelics, it also created feelings of warmth and empathy towards others, as well as a euphoric "rush" as the drug's effects were first felt. Euphoria, energy, empathy: the perfect party drug. It even made the endlessly-repetitive beats of trance music sound good!

Ecstasy creates these effects by releasing serotonin in the brain and central nervous system. Serotonin is a naturally-occurring neurotransmitter – a chemical that sends messages round the brain – which helps regulate sleep, appetite, muscle contractions, intestinal movements and mood. (When people have clinical depression, we give them Selective Serotonin Reuptake Inhibitors (SSRIs), which help to increase the level of serotonin available to do its work.) Dopamine, a pleasure hormone, is also released, contributing to the sense of euphoria. Users start feeling the effects of the drug 30–60 minutes after taking a pill, and these effects

Drugs – without the hot air, David Nutt

peak after 1–2 hours. Some people prefer to buy the drug as a powder and snort it, which produces faster and more short-lived effects. In recent years this has probably become the most common form, as the purity of pills has decreased.

Does ecstasy kill?

The first widely-publicised deaths involving ecstasy were mostly young men, who died of dehydration and hyperthermia (abnormally high body temperature) after dancing for hours in badly ventilated clubs without drinking enough water. Alongside a certain amount of media hysteria, some very sensible public-health advice went out in response to this, and clubs began providing free water and chill-out rooms to help dancers cool down. Deaths from dehydration fell once this was understood by venues and clubbers.

Unfortunately, this advice didn't make it clear that drinking water was an antidote to the health risks of extreme physical exertion and sweating, not an antidote to the drug itself. As a result, the second wave of ecstasy-related deaths were mostly young women suffering from water intox-ication, which happens when a person drinks so much water that the sodium level in their blood plasma drops dangerously low. (The lower ratio of body water to body mass in women compared with men prob-ably explains why women are particularly at risk.) The most famous case was Leah Betts, who died just after her 18th birthday after taking two ec-stasy pills; when she began to feel ill she repeatedly drank large amounts of water, until her plasma sodium level was so low ("hyponatraemia") that this water was sucked into her brain cells by osmosis, causing her brain to swell. The increased pressure on her brain stem put her into a coma from which she never woke up. Again, a public health campaign about how much to drink (one pint an hour), how to drink it (sipping rather than gulping), and what to drink (sports drinks, or water with added salt), helped to reduce the number of deaths from this condition.

Alongside these more common causes of death, there have been the occasional cases of liver failure, kidney failure and sudden cessation of heartbeat. Serotonin is involved in regulating blood clotting, and some people have died from blood clots followed by uncontrolled bleeding. Ecstasy raises the heart rate and blood pressure, so heart attacks are not unknown, and some users have also suffered brain haemorrhages. These rare but fatal reactions are similar to allergies, and are probably the result of genetic susceptibilities or other underlying conditions – it's possible that one day we'll be able to test for particular genes that make these reactions more likely. Of course, these are all tragedies for the families involved, but they're considerably [†]less common than other allergies which can be fatal, such as peanut allergies.

What are the other harms of ecstasy?

As time went by and deaths became less common, the focus of research and public-health campaigns moved from the dangers of dying or long term physical damage, to concerns about ecstasy's psychological effects. In particular, a lot of research has looked at the possible harm it might do to serotonin nerve cells, a process called neurodegeneration. Studies which [†]gave rats and monkeys huge doses of the drug did find that it harmed their serotonin cells, but despite a concerted effort to replicate this in humans when it was being trialled for medical use, ecstasy has never been shown to cause neurodegeneration at normal doses.

Heavy users have been shown to have [†]a degree of cognitive impairment and memory loss, but this is mild and short term, and almost always improves once they stop taking ecstasy. It's hard to know with poly drug users how responsible any individual substance is for causing problems, and this impairment is probably caused by the other drugs and activities people indulge in under the influence of ecstasy, such as dancing for hours. An interesting study of [†]Mormon teenagers, who were taking ecstasy but no other drugs, and no alcohol, found no differences between their mental functioning and those who took no drugs at all.

Despite concerns that ecstasy might interfere in the long-term with our serotonin systems, [†]causing depression, studies that have looked at this haven't found a clinically significant link. Although heavy ecstasy

Drugs – without the hot air, David Nutt

users, particularly those with a specific genotype, score slightly worse on depression rating scales overall, even the worst affected weren't in the range for clinical depression. A recent trial of treating post-traumatic stress disorder (PTSD) with MDMA (ie ecstasy) has shown extremely encouraging results; as PTSD has a strong relationship with depression, it may be that ecstasy can be used to treat mood disorders. We simply don't know, because the research has never been done.

Ecstasy in the media

The media have an intense and often disproportionate interest in the harms of ecstasy, in large part because of how the drug was introduced into the UK. Ecstasy first appeared in dance venues in the USA in the early 1980s, and came to Europe after being used by thousands of clubbers in Ibiza in the summer of 1986. The drug had a profound impact on the genre of dance music, and soon large crowds were being pulled into clubs by the promise of the kind of euphoric trance music that sounded particularly good if you were high on ecstasy. Although extremely popular, this created †two new problems for the club owners. The first was that the dancers were inevitably followed by the criminal gangs who were providing the illegal drug everyone wanted to take; the second was that ecstasy users didn't drink much alcohol, which the dance clubs depended on for their profits. As clubs became too expensive to hire, event organisers started looking for spaces they could use without paying – open fields in summer and empty warehouses in winter. In the days before the internet, the "rave" or "free party" organizer would announce a meet-point over pirate radio, and then lead a convoy of cars to the secret location which they'd occupy for the duration of their party.

These parties did pose a genuine health and safety challenge: at big events, thousands of people were mixing large quantities of drugs, in remote locations that were difficult for the emergency services to reach if something went wrong, especially in the days before mobile phones. Although the users themselves were unlikely to be aggressive or behave antisocially, the drug dealers making money at the parties were sometimes violent, and this was extremely difficult to police. However, while these concerns were real, a lot of the pressure on the government to respond to "rave culture" derived from several other social issues which were then current, such as the protests against the Conservative road expansion programme, squatter and traveller rights, and hunt saboteurs. Since ecstasy was already illegal, John Major's government took the step of banning "free parties" in the Criminal Justice and Public Order Act of 1994, defining a rave as an event which played music with [†]"repetitive beats" in unlicensed venues. This essentially forced dancers back into clubs which either charged high entrance fees or relied on clubbers consuming a lot of alcohol. In fact, the only significant dip or levelling out in Britain's steady increase in alcohol consumption over the past five decades was from the end of the 1980s to the mid-1990s [†](Figure 2.1), because so many people switched to ecstasy during that period.

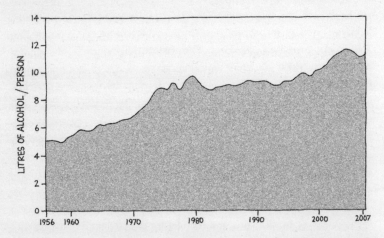

Figure 2.1: Rise in estimated alcohol consumption (in litres of alcohol per person over the age of 14).

The result of this social and legal background was that ecstasy became a "story" for the media, associated with anti-government protest and youthful counter-culture. As a result, there has been the systematic [†]over-reporting of ecstasy-related problems compared with other drugs,

Drugs – without the hot air, David Nutt

giving the impression that ecstasy is more harmful than it actually is. An enlightening study of the Scottish press from 1990 to 1999 compared newspaper reports of drug deaths with official coroners' data. It found that media interest varied considerably depending on the drug involved. Out of 265 deaths from paracetamol, the media reported only one, but a third of deaths from amphetamine (13 out of 36) made it into the news. Over the same time period, there were 28 deaths from ecstasy, 26 of which were reported – a far higher proportion than any other drug.

Of course, only stories that fit with the narrative that "ecstasy is bad for you" receive this kind of media coverage. An example of the contrast between the reaction to "good" news and "bad" news about the drug took place in the USA in 2002. A scientist called George Ricaurte published a †paper in *Science*, which claimed to have found new evidence that ecstasy caused "severe dopaminergic neurotoxicity" in monkeys. As this effect hadn't been found in previous studies at low doses, this surprised many other scientists in the field, but if true it could mean that recreational ecstasy users were putting themselves at risk of developing diseases like Parkinson's in later life. Ricaurte's study was widely reported at the time, especially as the Reducing Americans' Vulnerability to Ecstasy (RAVE) Bill was going through Congress at the time. Then, in September 2003, Ricaurte published a †formal retraction of his paper: somehow, two vials of drugs had got mixed up, and the neurotoxicity he had found had actually been caused by methamphetamine (crystal meth). The retraction received almost no attention from the media. "Ecstasy causes Parkinson's" is a story, whereas "ecstasy is no more harmful than we previously thought" isn't worth reporting.

In fact, rather than causing Parkinson's, ecstasy may actually be †an effective treatment for controlling its debilitating tremor. If the research that is currently underway into this topic delivers positive results, this will be evidence of yet another therapeutic use of the drug, alongside its beneficial effects in reducing anxiety in terminal cancer patients and in treating post-traumatic stress disorder (see box on page 24). These breakthroughs rarely make headlines, and indeed ecstasy currently has no officially approved medicinal uses at all.

All illegal drugs have both a Class, which determines the penalties for possession and supply, and a Schedule, which determines how they are regulated for medicinal use. Ecstasy is in Schedule I, which means the government does not recognise any medicinal uses, despite mounting evidence that it is much more effective than current drugs for several chronic, treatment-resistant disorders. Part of the reason ecstasy remains in an inappropriate Schedule is because the media are so obsessed with its harmful qualities, making it very difficult for politicians to consider any change in its classification. When the ACMD recommended that ecstasy be downgraded to Class B in 2008, [†]the government made it clear that no matter what the evidence indicated, they were not going to consider any reduction in the Class A status of Ecstasy.

Ecstasy: a moral issue

Ecstasy is a harmful drug – in no way should this chapter be interpreted as saying anything different. But how harmful? As harmful as drinking five pints of beer? As harmful as getting on a motorbike? David Spiegel-halter, a professor of risk communication, has calculated that taking an ecstasy pill is [†]as dangerous as riding a motorbike for about 6 miles or a push-bike for 20 miles. These sorts of comparisons are useful because they can help people make choices about their behaviour based on a realistic assessment of the risks. Politicians, however, are often highly resistant to them.

When Jacqui Smith called me to ask me to apologise for my equasy editorial (page 13), we had the following exchange:

Jacqui Smith: *You can't compare harms from a legal activity with an illegal one.*

Me: *Why not?*

Jacqui Smith: *Because one's illegal.*

Me: *Why is it illegal?*

Jacqui Smith: *Because it's harmful.*

Drugs – without the hot air, David Nutt

Me: *Don't we need to compare harms to determine if it should be illegal?*

Jacqui Smith: *You can't compare harms from a legal activity with an illegal one.*

It's not the only time I've had this circular conversation with an MP. This illegality logic loophole stems from the same philosophical starting point as the "War on Drugs" (which we'll look at in more detail later on). In our exchange, Jacqui Smith wanted to assert that drug use was an entirely different category of activity, incomparable to anything else. In this world-view, taking certain drugs in certain sorts of ways is not just harmful but *immoral*; it follows that policy-makers aren't interested in measuring harm – because they would want to eradicate this kind of drug use even if it wasn't doing any harm at all. This in turn leads to an emphasis on policies to reduce the *total number of users*, rather than the *total amount of harm*.

This is problematic for a number of reasons. For a start, it shoots policy-makers in the foot somewhat, since it's [†]not at all clear that governments are especially influential on whether or not someone *tries* a drug, because experimentation is largely determined by social norms and cultural trends. (Government policies can, however, be very influential on whether or not an individual is *harmed* by a drug.) In addition, if policies that aim for total abstinence do meet with some success, this will primarily be among casual users (who will find it easiest to give up altogether), rather than the heavy users and addicts who suffer the most harm. If we focused solely on reducing the prevalence of alcohol use, for example, it's the 30 million British drinkers who stay within the recommended daily limits who would be most likely to become teetotal, if any did at all. It would be absurd to aim an alcohol-harm-reduction strategy at those who suffer the least harm, rather than trying to help the 10 million hazardous drinkers to reduce their intake.

In addition, the focus on reducing prevalence can end up undermining measures that *are* shown to reduce harm, in case these measures "encourage" people to experiment with drugs. A case in point was the [†]Reducing Americans' Vulnerability to Ecstasy (RAVE) Act which became law in the USA in 2003, supported by the misleading evidence from Ricaurte's neurotoxicity study. The Act put more responsibility on venues to curb illegal drug use on their premises, citing features such as selling bottled water and providing chill out rooms as evidence that a venue was catering to the needs of ecstasy-users.

†Critics of the legislation pointed out that these were precisely the public-health measures that had helped to bring down the number of ecstasy-related deaths from dehydration, and that if venues ceased to provide water or spaces to cool down out of fear of prosecution this could lead to a rise in deaths.   As I said above, there is no clear relationship between policies like the RAVE Act and levels of use, so the most likely effect would be that young people would continue to take ecstasy in the same numbers under less safe conditions. But even if a small number of people were dissuaded from using ecstasy by the RAVE Act, it's perverse that this would be charted up as a "success" if the harm done to users had increased overall.

Why measuring drug harms frightens politicians

The problems of the RAVE Act illustrate why governments are so nervous about measuring drug harms. Being "tough on drugs" requires governments to reduce prevalence, but prevalence alone is the wrong thing to measure – it's only one factor among many that make up the total effect of drugs on society; †Figure 2.2 shows the USA's estimated total costs in billions of dollars of legal and illegal drugs, and of some other major causes of health problems. Prevalence does have a relationship with harm, and reducing use (particularly among specific target groups such as teenagers) might play a role in an effective harm-reduction strategy, but it is also the area where we are most in the dark about what works. What's more, not only are policies aimed at reducing prevalence unlikely to work, they often cause more harm than good in other ways. Measuring these other sorts of harm would discredit governmental policies, so often the data isn't collected and this kind of analysis isn't done.

Drug harms are very complex. My comparison of ecstasy with horse-

Drugs – without the hot air, David Nutt

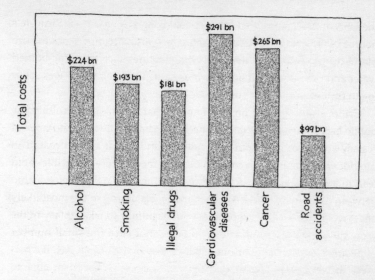

Figure 2.2: Estimated total economic costs of legal and illegal drugs, compared with other major causes of health problems, in the USA.

riding was a back-of-the-envelope calculation, trying to get a rough idea of the scale of the harms caused by each activity rather than precise figures. Even so, I had to take into account several different types of harm, some of which were to individuals (such as deaths and addiction) and some of which were to other people (such as crime and economic cost). This was not complete and I may have missed out some important dimensions – for example, I didn't take into account the harm done to the horses themselves, who often †die in big races and jumping events. It's important that our measurements are comprehensive, or a policy which reduces harm in one area might be increasing the negative consequences somewhere else in the system. In the next chapter we'll look at one way to think about harm much more systematically, comparing drugs with each other across a range of different criteria.

Of course, if you truly see illicit drug use as a moral problem, then it doesn't matter if drug users cause themselves harm, because they took a risk and any negative consequences are their own fault. However, this is illogical, since the level of risk in taking drugs is about the same as in everyday activities like horseriding, which aren't seen as immoral, and good policies for horse-riding involve helmets and safety-conscious riding rather than stopping people getting on horseback. It is also inhumane, going against the principles of universal healthcare that the UK's National Health Service was founded upon, where even self-inflicted illness deserves compassionate treatment. And it is misinformed, failing to understand how public health works. The huge improvements in the nation's health we have seen over the past century have come about precisely because we started treating *everybody*: diseases are infectious, and everybody benefits from helping those at most at risk of contracting and passing them on. Drug users are part of society, and when we treat them as such the outcomes improve for everybody, including non-drug users.

My comparison of horse-riding with ecstasy began when I treated a patient with brain damage – a woman you could see as being "responsible" for her condition, in that if she'd never got on horseback she wouldn't have suffered the injury. Yet the *Daily Mail* would never run a headline blaming her for her condition, or calling on the government to put horse riders in prison because of the burden they place on society. Compassionate treatment for her and her children helped to relieve some of the worst of their suffering, and this kind of care for vulnerable people is seen as a marker of a civilised society in other areas of health. We should apply this kind of thinking to drug use, and start seriously trying to reduce harm rather than prevalence alone.

Ecstasy and post-traumatic stress disorder

Post-traumatic stress disorder (PTSD) is a condition that sometimes occurs after a catastrophic life event or traumatic experience, such as witnessing a murder or being mugged at gunpoint. The patient suffers flashbacks, anxiety, fear, and nightmares, and may do anything to avoid reliving the experience – by refusing to leave the house, for example.

Drugs – without the hot air, David Nutt

PTSD is surprisingly common – [†]7.7 million people in Europe suffer from it each year. It's very disabling and associated with high rates of self harm and suicide. Rates are especially high among soldiers, who are far more likely to experience violent events than civilians – a study in 2004 found [†]18% of soldiers returning from Iraq and Afghanistan had PTSD, and more die from suicide than from combat.

The best treatment is trauma-focused therapy, where the memories are recalled in a safe setting, so the patient can learn that they're not in danger any more, and overcome the fear of them. However, a problem with this approach is that re-engaging with memories of trauma may be too stressful to contemplate. There are a number of "traditional" drugs used to treat it, such as benzodiazepines (page 217) and SSRIs (page 221), but the condition is often treatment-resistant and can last for years.

If we wanted to invent a drug especially designed to help enhance trauma-focused therapies, it would have the following qualities:

1. Be short-acting enough for a single session of therapy.
2. Have no significant dependency issues.
3. Be non-toxic at therapeutic doses.
4. Reduce feelings of depression that accompany PTSD.
5. Increase feelings of closeness between the patient and therapist.
6. Raise arousal to enhance motivation for therapy.
7. Paradoxically, increase relaxation and reduce hyper-vigilance.
8. Stimulate new ways of thinking to explore entrenched problems.

Ecstasy has all these qualities when used in a clinical setting, and is extremely effective. A recent study of subjects with chronic, treatment-resistant PTSD resulted in an [†]83% success rate – 10 out of 12 subjects essentially no longer had the disorder after just two sessions of ecstasy-assisted psychotherapy (Figure 2.3). The study also found no adverse drug-related events or neurocognitive effects. Of course, rare "allergic reactions" to the drug are still possible, but all medical treatments are potentially harmful – if the risk is small and the benefit is large, then the treatment can be justified. Within a clinical setting and under medical supervision, bad reactions to ecstasy are almost unknown, and the benefit is relieving otherwise unremitting PTSD.

This risk/benefit ratio looks pretty good to me, and to most others in the medical profession, and most importantly, to the patients themselves. We allow cancer patients to choose to be treated with highly toxic drugs which may damage their hearts or livers, or cause secondary cancers later in life if they survive the initial treatment, and we also allow surgical patients to face considerable risks of death. Yet because of ecstasy's legal status thousands of people suffering from PTSD aren't allowed to make a far less risky medical decision for themselves.

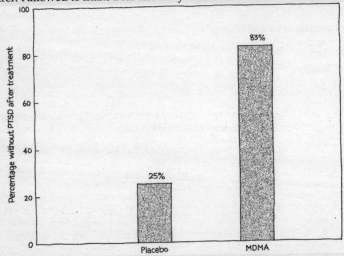

Figure 2.3: Comparison of placebo and MDMA (ecstasy) in treating post-traumatic stress disorder, showing percentage of patients who no longer had PTSD after treatment. (Higher is better.)

Drugs – without the hot air, David Nutt

Notes

Page

9 10 people die while horse riding• *Equasy: an overlooked addiction with implications for the current debate on drug harms*, David Nutt, Journal of Psychopharmacology 23 (1), 2009

9 100 road traffic accidents• As above.

10 research from the National Spinal Injuries Centre at Stoke Mandeville hospital• *Hazards of horse-riding as a popular sport*, JR Silver and JM Lloyd Parry, Br J Sp Med; 25(2), 1991

10 2 million riding episodes a year•Assume 200,000 riders, each of whom rides 10 times a year for an hour each time, say.

10 ecstasy as the sole cause of death for 10–17 people a year, and it's mentioned on the death certificates of 33–50 others• *MDMA ("ecstasy"): a review of its harms and classification under the Misuse of Drugs Act 1971*, ACMD, URL-8, February 2008

11 2,000 serious but non-fatal injuries from ecstasy every year• As above.

11 1,000 of those who seek specialist treatment for drug dependence every year say it's the main drug they're abusing• As above.

11 Melanie Reid• *Horse Sense*, Melanie Reid, *The Times*, March 12th 2011

12 60 million tablets• *MDMA ("ecstasy"): a review of its harms and classification under the Misuse of Drugs Act 1971*, ACMD, URL-8, February 2008

12 acute•An *acute* condition is one with a rapid onset, or a short duration, or both. (Whereas in normal speech "acute" is often used to mean "severe", in the medical sense you can have a condition that is acute but *not* severe.)

    Chronic is the opposite of acute – meaning a condition that lasts a long time. (Again, you can have a condition that is chronic but not severe.)

13 editorial• *Equasy: an overlooked addiction with implications for the current debate on drug harms*, David Nutt, Journal of Psychopharmacology 23 (1), 2009

13 *"makes light of a serious problem*,• *Drugs Adviser Criticised by Smith*, BBC news, February 9th 2009

13 *"completely incomparable"*, and that I was in the *"wrong job"*.• As above, the MP in question was Laurence Robertson, MP for Tewkesbury.

16 less common than other allergies which can be fatal, such as peanut allergies• *Drugs drive politicians out of their minds*, New Scientist, URL-9, February 11th 2009

16 gave rats and monkeys huge doses of the drug• *MDMA ("ecstasy"): a review of its harms and classification under the Misuse of Drugs Act 1971*, ACMD, URL-8, February 2008

16 a degree of cognitive impairment and memory loss• *Dancing hot on Ecstasy: physical activity and thermal comfort ratings are associated with the memory and other psychobiological problems reported by recreational MDMA users*, AC Parrott, J Rodgers, T Buchanan et al. *Human Psychopharmacology: Clinical and Experimental* 21: 285–98, 2006

16 Mormon teenagers• *The harmful health effects of recreational ecstasy: a systematic review of observational evidence*, G Rogers et al, Health Technology Assessment, January 2009

16 causing depression• *MDMA ("ecstasy"): a review of its harms and classification under the Misuse of Drugs Act 1971*, ACMD, URL-8, February 2008

17 two new problems for the club owners• *The Hacienda: How Not to Run a Club*, Peter Hook, Simon & Schuster Ltd, 2009

18 "repetitive beats"• *Powers in relation to raves*, Criminal Justice and Public Order Act, URL-10, 1994

18 (Figure 2.1)• *Popular intoxicants: what lessons can be learned from the last 40 years of alcohol and cannabis regulation?*, Ruth Weissenborn and David J Nutt, Journal of Psychopharmacology, September 17th 2011. Sources: *British Beer and Pub Association Statistical Handbook 2008*; Institute of Alcohol Studies Factsheet *Trends in the affordability of alcohol in the UK*, 2008.

18 over-reporting of ecstasy-related problems compared with other drugs• *Distorted? a quantitative exploration of drug fatality reports in the popular press*, Alasdair JM Forsyth, International Journal of Drug Policy (12), 2001

19 paper in *Science*• *Severe dopaminergic neurotoxicity in primates after a common recreational dose regimen of MDMA*, George Ricaurte, Science, September 26th 2002

19 formal retraction of his paper• *Retraction: Severe dopaminergic neurotoxicity in primates after a common recreational dose regimen of MDMA*, George Ricaurte, Science, September 12th 2003

19 an effective treatment for controlling its debilitating tremor• *MDMA ("ecstasy"): a review of its harms and classification under the Misuse of Drugs Act 1971*, ACMD, URL-8, February 2008

20 the government made it clear that no matter what the evidence indicated• House of Commons, Minutes of Evidence, Science and Technology Committee, URL-160.

20 as dangerous as riding a motorbike for about 6 miles or a push-bike for 20 miles• *Cambridge Ideas – Professor Risk*, David Spiegelhalter, URL-11, December 10th 2009

21 not at all clear that governments are especially influential on whether or not someone *tries* a drug• *Drugs Policy - Lessons learnt and options for the future*, Mike Trace, URL-12, February 23rd 2011

21 Reducing Americans' Vulnerability to Ecstasy (RAVE) Act• *RAVE Act*, US Senate, URL-13, 2003. In fact the original RAVE Act was never passed, but the Illicit Drug Anti-Proliferation Act, which incorporated much of the orginal RAVE Act was enacted in April 2003.

22 Critics of the legislation• *Innocent club owners, young people vulnerable under rapidly moving "Rave" Bill*, Drug Policy Alliance, URL-14, July 11th 2002

22 Figure 2.2• *Recent Findings on the Economic Impacts of Substance Abuse*, Henrick Harwood, URL-179, presented to American Psychological Association, Science Leadership Conference, October 23, 2011

23 die in big races and jumping events• *Race Horse Deaths*, URL-15, accessed December 10th 2011

25 7.7 million people in Europe suffer from it each year• *The size and burden of mental disorders and other disorders of the brain in Europe 2010*, URL-164, HU Wittchen, F Jacobi et al, European Neuropsychopharmacology (21) 655–679, 2011

25 18% of soldiers• *Combat duty in Iraq and Afghanistan, mental health problems, and barriers to care*, Charles W Hoge et al, The New England Journal of Medicine (351), 2004

25 83% success rate• *The safety and efficacy of 3,4-methylenedioxymethamphetamine-assisted psychotherapy in subjects with chronic, treatment-resistant post-traumatic stress disorder: the first randomized controlled pilot study*, Michael Mithoefer et al, Journal of Psychopharmacology 25 (4) 439–452, 2010

3 How can we measure the harms done by drugs?

Why measure?

When the UK's Misuse of Drugs Act became law in the UK in 1971, it put a range of drugs previously controlled under the Poisons Act into three Classes: A, B and C. As discussed in chapter 1, a drug's classification was intended to reflect the harm it did, with greater penalties for possession and supply of more dangerous substances. This legal structure was intended to be flexible, with drugs moving up and down the Class system as new evidence emerged. In practice, there have never been clear or transparent justifications for the legal Class a drug has received, and there has been very little movement between Classes – especially very little downward movement – in the light of new evidence. The Advisory Council on the Misuse of Drugs (ACMD) was also created by the Act, to examine the science, and produce recommendations for the government to follow.

In effect the ACMD was formed to take party politics out of drug-harm assessments, because it was known that politicians liked to vie with each other as to who could be the "hardest" on drugs: even in the 1970s, this was seen as an easy way to score political points and gain media support. So a group of experts were given the responsibility for drug assessment – in much the same way as the Bank of England has since been given responsibility for setting interest rates. And for many years this worked. When the UK was facing a major problem with HIV/AIDS arising from injected heroin use, the ACMD approached the then Prime Minister Mrs Thatcher and †recommended needle exchange programmes. Even though this conflicted with her political philosophy she agreed to go with the ACMD's recommendations, and the UK ended up with one of the lowest rates of HIV among injecting drug users in Europe. This made the UK a beacon of preventative policy for the world.

When I first joined the ACMD in 1998, I thought that, broadly, government policy was going along the right lines. As time went by, however, I began to see that there were serious problems with the government's approach. I became frustrated with politicians' almost-religious aversion to comparing the risks posed by legal and illegal activities, illustrated so clearly in the response to my equasy editorial (page 13). I began to question whether criminalisation was ever an effective or appropriate moral response to drug use (which I'll talk about in more detail in chapter 15). But above all, in terms of my specific role in the ACMD, I became deeply unhappy with the way the government was ignoring the recommendations we were producing about the Classes that should be allocated to certain drugs, notably ecstasy, mushrooms and cannabis. The Misuse of Drugs Act may not be a perfect piece of legislation, but at least the government could use it rationally, and do what the Act required by listening to the expert Advisory Council it set up.

I started to think about the whole purpose of classification. Clearly, some drugs are more harmful than others, and people should have a broad understanding of the risks if they choose to take them. Politicians sometimes invoke the precautionary principle to argue that, if we're not completely sure if something might do harm, we should put it in as high a Class as possible. However, this may be unwise as it can have perverse consequences. There was a very sad tale a few years ago of a †young girl in the Shetland Islands who wanted to try cannabis, but could only get hold of heroin and died of an overdose; if cannabis and heroin are in the same Class, indicating that they pose the same sorts of risks, this kind of tragedy may happen more often. More generally, people aren't stupid, and have access to other sources of information about drugs apart from the government. If the other evidence and the government response don't seem to add up, it undermines public confidence in what the government is doing and makes giving a credible educational message impossible.

Having different categories of drugs is sensible. Almost no ordinary member of the public is going to read long scientific reports, and having a simple way to assess relative harmfulness would be useful for a lot of people, regardless of what criminal sanctions are attached to which Class. If a drug's position in the Class system was actually determined by how harmful it is on a number of different measures, then people might understand the risks they were taking better, and even choose to take substances in lower Classes which will do them less damage.

Measuring drug harms poses many challenges. Could we find a way of *measuring* the harms done by drugs, based on an evidence-based assessment of the damage that they actually caused? What if we included substances that are currently legal, and thought seriously about how the harms they cause compared with illegal drugs – what Class would alcohol and tobacco be? And how could we make this *transparent*, so that people trusted the information we were giving them, and *flexible*, so that drugs could be upgraded or downgraded as we learned more about them? I've spent much of the last fifteen years trying to answer these sorts of questions.

Sixteen different sorts of harm

Measuring drug harms is a complicated process. There are lots of different sorts of harm to consider – deaths each year, chronic illness, mental-health problems, social problems like crime and violence, etc. Some drugs are particularly harmful in some areas but not in others; interestingly, this balance can change over time as patterns of use develop and new trends emerge. Our knowledge can be quite patchy, particularly about new drugs as they appear on the streets. A big part of the challenge of measuring drug harms is how we can think about lots of different sorts of harm at the same time.

My first attempt to compare drugs harms was in [†]a paper I co-wrote in 2007, where we looked at 9 different sorts of harm – 3 physical, 3 social and 3 associated with dependence. We received a lot of constructive criticism, and once we had taken on board our critics' comments we came up with a comprehensive list of 16 criteria of harm, 9 to users, and 7 to others. By this time I had been sacked by the government and had set up the ISCD, so [†]my second paper, published in 2010, was under those auspices, although [†]the initial development of the 16 criteria was with the ACMD. These 16 criteria were:

Harms to users

1. *Drug-specific mortality* – death from poisoning. We measure how poisonous a substance is by comparing the amount needed to give psychoactive effects and the amount that would be fatal; this gives a *safety ratio*. For example, alcohol's safety ratio is 10. If 2 units of alcohol are enough to have a psychoactive effect on a small female, 20 units will put her into a lethal coma. Some substances rarely if ever cause death by overdose – cannabis and LSD, for example.

2. *Drug-related mortality.* This includes deaths from chronic illnesses caused by drug-taking, such as cancers, and associated behaviours and activities. For example, injecting puts users at risk of hepatitis and HIV, and dangerous driving under the influence of a drug or drink causes road traffic accidents. Sometimes specific and related causes overlap: it may be an overdose of heroin that finally kills an addict, but the chronic health problems from the lifestyle will have weakened their cardiovascular system, making the person less likely to survive.

3. *Drug-specific harm.* Any physical damage (short of death) specifically caused by the drug – eg alcohol-related cirrhosis, tobacco-related lung disease (emphysema), cocaine nose, ketamine bladder.

4. *Drug-related harm.* Damage from drug-related activities and behaviours, short of death: viruses and infections, accidents, non-fatal road traffic accidents.

5. *Dependence.* We discuss the concept of addiction in chapter 8.

6. *Drug-specific impairment of mental functioning.* How far being intoxicated on the drug impairs judgement, which may lead to risky behaviours, including unprotected sex as well as drunk or drugged driving.

7. *Drug-related impairment of mental functioning.* While the previous criterion refers to the effects of intoxication, drug-related impairment of mental functioning refers to the psychological effects that continue once the drug has left the body. Heavy use of some drugs is associated with psychotic symptoms, depression, memory loss, increased aggression, and anhedonia (an inability to feel pleasure). Addiction also often leads to depression from the stress and unpleasantness of being a drug addict.

8. *Loss of tangibles.* Losing your job, your income, your possessions or your home, because of drug use.

9. *Loss of relationships.* People might lose friends or family because of their behaviour while intoxicated – being aggressive or reclusive – or because they are addicted and engage in compulsive behaviour, such as stealing from people they know to fund their habit.

Harms to others

10. *Injury.* Taking drugs usually impairs motor control and judgement, increasing the likelihood of an incident that damages someone else. This might be accidental, such as road traffic accidents, or deliberate, like domestic violence, both of which are hugely influenced by alcohol.

11. [†]*Crime* outside of the Misuse of Drugs Act (see endnote). Drug-related crime largely falls into two categories: (a) acquisitive crime to fund a drug habit, and (b) crime committed when judgement is impaired while under the influence, such as burglary and vandalism.

12. *Economic cost.* This includes workdays lost because people are taking or recovering from drugs, the amount of police time spent dealing with associated crime, and the cost to the NHS.

13. *Impact on family life.* As with loss of relationships, drugs may have a bad effect on family life because of the behaviour (particularly aggression) of family members while under the influence, or because of the compulsive behaviour of addicts. Includes child neglect.

Drugs – without the hot air, David Nutt

14. *International damage.* Although our main focus was on the UK, we knew we needed to factor-in harms on an international level. These include: the huge collateral damage of the War on Drugs; the brutality of the international drug barons, who are making billions from the illicit trade and have killed 25,000 people in Mexico alone; and the carbon emissions and other environmental effects due both to the drug manufacturers and the measures taken against them.

15. *Environmental damage.* Drug production can pollute local areas with toxic or flammable chemicals. Used needles and broken bottles can make local parks no-go areas for children, while noisy and aggressive behaviour also degrades the environment.

16. *Decline in reputation of the community.* Heavy drug use can stigmatise particular social groups and turn neighbourhoods into "no go" zones. Certain drugs, especially crack, are notorious for this.

The harms to the user would be considered purely on an individual level: what's the average amount of harm experienced by somebody who takes this drug? The harms to others, on the other hand, would be considered on a population level: given the total levels of consumption of this drug in the UK, how much harm do we suffer as a society? Both these dimensions of harm are important, and approaching them in this way allowed us to consider them simultaneously while also keeping them distinct.

Multi-criteria decision analysis

Another criticism of the 2007 paper was that we calculated the final score of harm by giving each factor the same weight, when in fact some of them might be more important than others. One of the people who approached us after reading our paper was Professor Larry Phillips, from the LSE (London School of Economics), an expert in †Decision Conferencing. He offered to help us design a new process for evaluating drug harms, using multi-criteria decision analysis.

Multi-criteria decision analysis (MCDA) is a technique often used in situations where a decision needs to take into account different *sorts* of information, and where there are so many dimensions that conclusions can't easily be drawn from simple discussion. MCDA breaks down an issue into different criteria, and then compares those criteria with each other to assess their relative importance. These criteria can include both objective measures and subjective value judgements, and can incorporate an element of uncertainty.

†Larry Phillips had previously worked on a big public consultation about the options for disposing of nuclear waste. Experts and members of the public considered different criteria, such as cost, safety, and the impacts on future generations, and then thought about how important each of these criteria was. This created a model which could be tested under different scenarios and with different interest groups; in the case of the nuclear consultation, they found that it needed quite significant changes in the weight given to different criteria for the most popular options for nuclear-waste storage to change. Since the model was very stable, even across interest groups as diverse as the nuclear industry and Greenpeace, it gave a great deal of legitimacy to the final decision. It was also very transparent: by making clear which parts of a decision are based on factual evidence and which parts are based on subjective value judgements, it's much easier to understand how a conclusion has been drawn or a decision has been made.

The expert panel

The panel we assembled to consider the 16 criteria of harm consisted of four professionals with different fields of expertise in working with drug users and in drugs research, as well as myself, plus many specialists from other areas. Five of us had formerly been part of the ACMD and one, criminologist Fiona Measham, was on the ACMD at the time we conducted the MCDA.

The panel included five experts in addiction:

- Colin Drummond, Professor of Addiction Psychiatry at the Institute of Psychiatry (IoP). He has spent much of his career studying alcohol problems, and chairs the group within the National Insti-

Drugs – without the hot air, David Nutt

tute for Clinical Excellence (NICE), which develops guidelines for managing harmful alcohol use and alcohol dependence.

- John Marsden, Reader in Addictive Behaviour at the IoP, who specialises in behavioural and pharmacological therapies for drug addiction.
- Penny Schofield, a GP who has written guidelines on methadone substitution treatment, and was formerly on the clinical team at the National Treatment Agency.
- Tim Williams, Consultant Psychiatrist in Drug Addiction. Tim studies the biological basis for addiction and risk factors for sudden death in drug users.
- Adam Winstock, Senior Lecturer in Addiction at the IoP, who specialises in improving the health outcomes of treatments for drug addiction by increasing the addicts' understanding of their own treatment.

We had two experts in drug issues relating to young people:

- Patrick Hargreaves, Durham County Council Drugs and Alcohol Adviser, who has developed promising new approaches to drugs education.
- Eric Carlin, who specialises in prevention and early intervention in drug use in young people.

The panel included two chemists:

- Les King, a former forensic scientist and adviser to the Department of Health and the European Monitoring Centre for Drugs and Drug Addiction.
- John Ramsey, a forensic scientist whose company, TicTac, provides the database for the visual identification of drugs used by the police and pharmaceutical industry.

Our other five experts came from a range of backgrounds:

- Phil Delgarno, a psychologist based at Glasgow Caledonian University, who studies drug use in its social context.

- Martin Frischer, Senior Lecturer at the University of Keele, who conducted some of the key research into the link between cannabis and schizophrenia that informed the ACMD's 2008 cannabis report.
- Fiona Measham, Reader in Criminology at the University of Lancaster, who specialises in emerging drug trends; chairs the ACMD's polysubstance group.
- Jeremy Sare, ex-secretary to the ACMD, and journalist who writes extensively on drugs and drugs policy.
- Nicola Singleton, Director of Policy and Research at the UK Drugs Policy Commission, who has conducted research into the enforcement of drugs policies by the police and criminal justice system.

Which drugs did the expert panel consider?

Stimulants:

- Amphetamine (Class B): pills or powder, mostly taken by clubbers.
- Methamphetamine (Class A): smokable crystal form of amphetamine, not common in the UK.
- Anabolic steroids (Class C): pills or powder, used to build up body mass.
- Khat: a legal leaf which is chewed, mostly used by people from the Middle East and East Africa.
- Mephedrone (Class B) pills or powder, popular with clubbers.
- Cocaine (Class A): powder, which is usually snorted.
- Crack (Class A): smokable crystal form of cocaine.
- Butane (legal): gas that can be inhaled, popular with teenagers.
- Tobacco (legal): usually smoked in cigarettes.

Depressants:

- Alcohol (legal): comes in drinks of different strengths.
- Benzodiazepines (Class C): a type of sleeping pills, mostly available on prescription (eg Valium).

Drugs – without the hot air, David Nutt

- Ketamine (Class C): powder which is snorted, or liquid which is injected, popular with clubbers.
- Cannabis (Class B) solid resin or leaves of plant, which are smoked or eaten; the most widely-used illegal drug in the world.
- GHB (Class C): powder which is usually dissolved in liquid and drunk, with similar effects to alcohol.

Opioids:

- Heroin (Class A): brown solid which can be smoked or "cooked up" into a liquid and injected.
- Methadone (Class A): pharmacological substitute for heroin; usually drunk as a liquid.
- Buprenorphine (Class C): pharmacological substitute for heroin; comes as a pill.

Empathogens and psychedelics:

- Ecstasy (Class A): pills or powder containing MDMA which produce feelings of energy and euphoria, popular with clubbers.
- LSD (Class A): liquid (on blotting paper) which causes psychedelic experiences in very small doses.
- Mushrooms (Class A): eaten whole or brewed as tea, and causing psychedelic experiences.

Rating the drugs

The first step of the MCDA process was to rate the 20 drugs according to each of the criteria. Let's take [†]drug-related mortality as an example. (Recall, we defined this as death caused by illnesses caused by drug-taking and associated behaviour and activities.) Looking across the drugs we decided that heroin was the worst for this criterion, mostly because of the spread of blood-borne viruses, and health problems associated with addiction and deprivation. Heroin was given a score of 100. The only drug that we thought caused no drug-related mortality was LSD, so this was given a score of 0. For drug-related mortality, this gave us a scale (Figure 3.1).

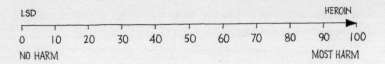

Figure 3.1: The 0–100 scale for drug-related mortality.

We then looked at the other 18 drugs and tried to estimate where they should go on the scale we just created. Tobacco, with its huge burden of fatal illnesses from cancers and heart attacks, was rated at 90. Magic mushrooms, which don't themselves kill, but sometimes get misidentified so people die from eating poisonous varieties, were given a score of 1. We based our estimates on our professional experience and expertise, discussing areas of disagreement until we came to an acceptable consensus. Figure 3.2 shows how we rated them all on the scale.

Our estimates of relative harm were given an objective quality through the discussion and debate that occurred during the rating process. We then corroborated our group judgements by [†]comparing our scores with measurements such as official statistics on drug-related deaths. We found strong relationships: for example, when we looked at fatality statistics and drug-specific mortality, the correlation was around 0.98, and looking at a USA survey on lifetime dependence and our own dependence scores we found a correlation of 0.95. (A perfect correlation is a score of 1.)

The rating process for other criteria did highlight a lack of objective data in many areas, particularly social harms. Here the expert group approach is the best we can do for now. While this is not perfect, it's important we make a start on a quantitative approach, and even approximate figures can give valuable insights, as well as highlighting where it's most important to concentrate future research efforts. If we wait until perfect data is available for everything, we paralyse the decision-making process and risk damaging or losing lives needlessly. MCDA exploits the fact that people are generally good at making relative judgements, particularly in well-informed groups, and using this method to measure harms means we don't have to wait until we have perfect information before we can make decisions that have clear and transparent justifica-

Drugs – without the hot air, David Nutt

tions. It's also very easy to incorporate new evidence as it comes to light. (See the section about ketamine on page 47 as an example.)

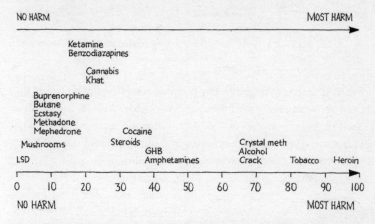

Figure 3.2: The 20 drugs examined by the independent panel, allocated to the 0–100 scale for drug-related mortality using multi-criteria decision analysis.

Weighting the scores

Having made scales (like those in Figure 3.2) for all 16 criteria, we then weighted them against each other. This had to take into account two things: how big a difference between 0 and 100 was, and how important we thought that difference was between each of the 16 measures. An analogy for how someone might weigh up different criteria like this in everyday life is if they're looking to buy a car. For most people, price is one of the biggest factors in choosing a vehicle, but if you went to a dealer and the difference between the most expensive and least expensive models was only £200, you would probably make your decision based on other factors like size or fuel efficiency. Context is important too – cost would probably be a much bigger issue if the price difference was £2,000, unless you were very rich and wouldn't notice a few grand here or there. Figure 3.3 illustrates the software we used to apply the different weightings when comparing the different drugs.

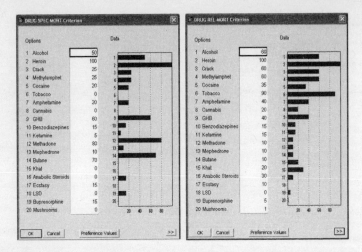

Figure 3.3: The software we used to assign different weights to the various drugs, here showing the resulting rankings for drug-specific, and drug-related, mortalities.

Of course, the weighting process involved judgements which can't be checked against objective measures. However, by experimenting with different weights we could see that the model was pretty stable. This process of changing the weightings in the model once it has been constructed is called "sensitivity analysis", and is a big advantage of MCDA. Our rankings were stable: even quite substantial changes did not affect the rank order. (In other words, the overall ranking was "insensitive" to minor changes – they did not significantly affect the result.) For example, the weight put on drug-specific mortality would have had to increase by 15 points before heroin overtook alcohol in first place as the most harmful drug overall. To appreciably affect the outcome would have required substantial changes like this in one or two areas, or lots of different smaller changes, so we were satisfied that the results were reliable.

Drugs – without the hot air, David Nutt

Results

Once we'd rated all the drugs and weighted the criteria, each drug got a final score out of 100. Alcohol came top with 72, followed by heroin and crack neck and neck at 55 and 54, with quite a big drop after that to methamphetamine on 33. At the very bottom were the empathogens and psychedelics, with ecstasy given a score of 9, and LSD and mushrooms on 7 and 6. [†]Figure 3.4 shows all 20 drugs ranked in order of total harms.

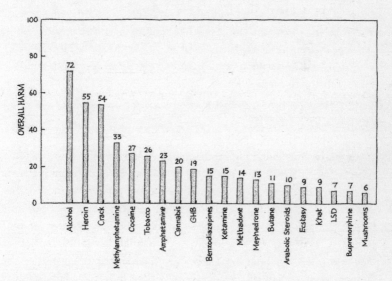

Figure 3.4: The 20 drugs considered in the ISCD's 2010 report, ranked by overall harm.

The first thing to note is how little relationship there is between a drug's current legal Class and the position we ranked it in. The top six substances did include four Class As, but there were also two drugs which are currently legal, which common sense says you'd expect to find among the least harmful. At the bottom end of the scale were another three Class As: ecstasy, LSD and mushrooms. In fact, when we compared legal Class and overall ranking, we found a correlation of 0.04 –

which means that there was effectively no relationship at all. By contrast, the correlation between this paper and my 2007 paper was 0.7, and the correlation with a similar Dutch study ranking drugs according to harm was around 0.8. Although these figures show that there wasn't perfect agreement across the three studies, they do indicate that we're all on a similar track, and in fact many of the differences can be attributed to different methodologies,

Note just how dangerous alcohol is – it was ranked as the fourth most harmful drug to the user, and most harmful drug to others (†Figure 3.5), making it top overall. Over half of its score came from economic cost, injury, family adversities and crime. While this is very worrying, we do at least have a lot of evidence about ways to reduce the harms done by alcohol, and implementing these should clearly be a priority in our policies relating to drugs.

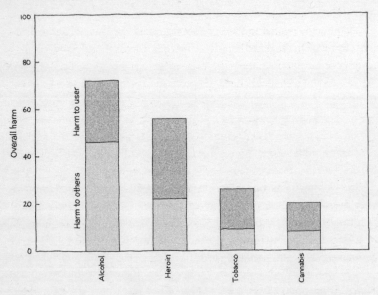

Figure 3.5: Four of the drugs considered in the ISCD's 2010 report, broken down by harm to user (top part of bar), and harm to others (bottom of bar).

Drugs – without the hot air, David Nutt

Limitations of the model

No model is perfect, and there were certain limitations to the approach we took.

First, we scored only the harms done by drugs, when in fact they all have benefits too (at least initially, otherwise no one would take them). Weighing up the benefits is already an established part of the argument for keeping alcohol and tobacco legal, since the jobs they provide and tax revenue they bring in offset their costs to an extent. A more nuanced model might try to think about both costs and benefits, and theoretically this would be very easy to do with MCDA, although politically it could be rather problematic.

Secondly, a lot of the harms done by drugs are affected by their availability and legal status, so ideally a model would be able to distinguish between harms directly related to the drug, and harms related to the legal control of a drug. A large part of the risk of overdose for heroin users, for example, is related to the fact that they can't get a clean and consistent supply. (On the other hand, the increasing availability of alcohol has certainly contributed to the huge surge in its harms over the last 50 years. There's no suggestion that heroin should be available on the supermarket shelves!)

Thirdly, most people are poly drug users, and our study considered only the impact of substances on their own. Certain drugs are more dangerous in combination – for example, alcohol with GHB, or alcohol with heroin – and we need more research into how they interact.

Finally, drug users are far from being a homogeneous group: there are very different patterns of use that can have very different harm profiles. A future model might be able to distinguish between different methods of taking drugs, between prescription and non-prescription users, and between addicts and non-addicts.

Critical reception

When the report came out, the headline *"Alcohol 'more harmful than heroin or crack'"* appeared on the front page of the *Guardian*, and it was widely reported across the British press and beyond. [†]The *Daily Mail* predictably called me a *"dangerous man"*; it said the policies I was advancing *"would be a disaster for our society"*. In fact I hadn't proposed any policies at all, but only a more rational approach to drug classification.

The government's response was interesting. Although the design of the decision analysis process had been publicly funded while I was still part of the ACMD, the Home Office's spokesperson said quite bluntly that they hadn't read the report, and continued: [†]*"our priorities are clear – we want to reduce drug use, crack down on drug-related crime and disorder and help addicts come off drugs for good."* This showed that much of the wrong-headedness of the Labour government in relation to drugs was likely to continue with the new coalition. Getting addicts off drugs for good is extremely difficult, as chapter 9 will show. Most drug-related crime is caused by addicts stealing to fund their habit, most drug-related disorder is related to people being drunk, and both addicts and drunks tend to be unresponsive to "crackdowns". And as I argued in chapter 1, reducing drug use on its own is not a useful aim for drug policy: trying to shift the focus away from reducing prevalence to reducing harm was exactly why I wanted to measure drug harms in a more comprehensive way.

Conclusion

When we wrote the 2007 paper, our primary aim was to examine whether or not the classification of drugs under the Misuse of Drugs Act reflected the harms they caused. The resounding conclusion of both that paper, and our later one in 2010, was that it didn't. So, could we reconstruct a new classification system out of our results? This would obviously depend on what set of harms – to self or others – you were trying to reduce, but in terms of overall harm, alcohol, heroin and crack are clearly more harmful than all the others, so perhaps drugs with a score of 40 or more could be Class A, 39–20 could be Class B, 19–10 B Class C, and 9–1 Class D. How widely available these should be and what penalties they should entail is another conversation altogether, but classifying in this

Drugs – without the hot air, David Nutt

way would at least give a consistent public-health message.

In terms of the process, multi-criteria decision analysis seems to be a promising approach to dealing with the complex interwoven issues around drug harms. It can be re-run with different interest groups, particularly in the weighting stage, and it would be interesting to see how, for example, drug users and their families prioritised the different criteria compared with our expert panel. An ex-MP has talked about trying to get other MPs interested in the weighting process, and involving them in this way might help them think differently about what drug classification is for, and what their policies are trying to achieve.

All models have their limitations, but this 2010 one is more flexible and sophisticated than my 2007 version, and obviously far more grounded in evidence than the current Class A/B/C system. We welcome science-based criticism of the model, and we hope that it will be improved on in time, both by the ISCD and other groups and organisations. It's true that this isn't "pure" science, but it's "interpreting" science – putting it into a form that politicians and the public can understand. Our knowledge about drugs will never be complete, but in the meantime politicians need to make laws, and people have to make decisions about what drugs they take and in what way. We shouldn't let the "best be the enemy of the good", searching for the perfect evidence-based model before we change anything when our current classification system is clearly unfit for purpose.

Reviewing a drug's Class? The case of ketamine

†Ketamine was invented in 1963, as a substitute for phencyclidine, an anaesthetic agent. Ketamine is a powerful anaesthetic, and very safe because it depresses breathing very little and doesn't stop the gag reflex, but it is rarely used in mainstream medicine because of its psychoactive effects. It is commonly used on animals, which is why it is often referred to as "horse tranquilliser". The USA saw a certain amount of ketamine abuse after the Vietnam war where it was used in the combat zones. In the UK, until the 1990s recreational use of the drug was limited to a small

number of self-styled "psychonauts", who would inject medicinal supplies to explore the weird inner worlds that ketamine can reveal.

A new sort of abuse emerged in the 1990s, as the drug users associated with the dance scene started to manufacture their own ketamine as a white powder, or to buy it in from India in solution, mislabelled as "rosewater". It was legal and relatively cheap, and made a good "downer" at the end of a night on stimulants such as ecstasy and amphetamines; it was also often mixed with cocaine and snorted in a concoction known as CK1. The ACMD became concerned in the early 2000s, and recommended it become a Class C drug in its †2004 report, advice which was acted upon by the government in 2006. The report still thought that ketamine's dependence profile was low and that it would primarily be used in the poly drug setting: we thought the main harm it was doing was interacting with other substances, making intoxicated people less aware of their surroundings so they were more prone to accidents and misadventure. The scores our expert panel gave ketamine over the 16 criteria in our 2010 paper were largely based on our understanding of the drug from the ACMD's 2004 report.

In the intervening years however, new evidence had started to come to light, which was eventually written up in the ISCD's first drug report in 2010, about six months after we went through the decision analysis process. Two new trends were causing concern for drug workers and GPs: an increase in the number of people seeking help for ketamine dependence, and an increase in young people (especially young men) with urinary tract problems related to ketamine use, called "ketamine-induced ulcerative cystitis". This is a newly-identified condition, where the bladder goes into spasm and its wall thickens, resulting in a small bladder capacity. It's not entirely clear why ketamine has this effect, but one theory is that it activates the nerve fibres in the bladder, affecting its ability to expand and contract as it fills and empties. Symptoms include needing to pee frequently and urgently, incontinence, pain when peeing, and blood in the urine. In extreme cases it's irreversible, and patients need reconstruction or removal of the bladder altogether, resulting in the need for lifelong medical care. New evidence also emerged about kidney problems, abnormal liver function and severe abdominal pain ("k cramps") probably originating from the bladder. This new evidence showed that ketamine, especially when taken daily in high doses, is more harmful than we previously thought.

Had we known these facts while running the decision analysis, we might have rated it higher for both dependence and drug-specific damage. The advantage of the model is that we can experiment with changing things, and rerun it with different numbers. We can see that increasing its score on these two criteria by only 5 points makes it more harmful than benzodiazepines overall, but it takes a leap of nearly 40 points on these two criteria to bring its final score above that of GHB. So the rank order of the drugs remains pretty stable so long as it's only one or two criteria that need revision, and ketamine would be unlikely to move from Class C if that referred to drugs scoring between 10 and 19.

Notes
Page

30 recommended needle exchange programmes• *The role and basis of drug laws*, David Nutt, Prometheus, 2010

31 young girl in the Shetland Islands• *Estimating Drug Harms: A Risky Business?*, David Nutt, URL-2, October 10th 2009

32 a paper I co-wrote in 2007• *Development of a rational scale to assess the harm of drugs of potential misuse*, Nutt et al, Lancet, 2007

33 my second paper, published in 2010• *Drug harms in the UK: a multicriteria decision analysis*, David Nutt et al, ISCD, URL-16, November 1st 2010

33 the initial development of the 16 criteria• *Consideration of the use of Multi-Criteria Decision Analysis in drug harm decision making*, ACMD, URL-17, July 28th 2010

34 *Crime* outside of the Misuse of Drugs Act• We did not consider crimes directly related to the production, supply and possession of substances controlled under the Misuse of Drugs Act in this criterion, or anywhere in our analysis. Since part of our aim was to make a direct comparison between legal and illegal substances, it was felt that including the harms stemming directly from legal status would skew the calculation with Jacqui Smith's circular logic that we outlined in chapter 2 – because it is a crime to produce, supply or possess a substance it must be more harmful than a drug which can be obtained legally.

35 Decision Conferencing•See URL-182 for a description of decision conferencing.

36 Larry Phillips had previously worked on a big public consultation about the options for disposing of nuclear waste• *Committee on Radioactive Waste Management Public Lecture*, Larry Phillips, URL-18, October 11th 2006, a very informative and interesting podcast about Larry's work on the consultation, with the slides also available for download.

39 drug-related mortality• See *Development of a rational scale to assess the harm of drugs of potential misuse*, Nutt et al, Lancet, 2007, for more detail on how this is defined.

40 comparing our scores with measurements such as official statistics• *Improving Data Input in the MCDA Model Based on Evidence*, Y Mu, MSc Thesis LSE, 2010

43 Figure 3.4• *Drug harms in the UK: a multicriteria decision analysis*, David Nutt et al, ISCD, URL-16, November 1st 2010

44 Figure 3.5• *Drug harms in the UK: a multicriteria decision analysis*, as above.

46 The *Daily Mail* predictably called me a *"dangerous man"*; it said the policies I was advancing *"would be a disaster for our society"* • *Why doesn't this dangerous man come clean and admit he wants to legalise drugs?*, Stephen Glover, URL-19, November 3rd 2009

46 *"our priorities are clear – we want to reduce drug use, crack down on drug-related crime and disorder and help addicts come off drugs for good."*• *Alcohol "more harmful than heroin" says Prof David Nutt*, BBC news, URL-20, Nov 1st 2010

47 Ketamine was invented in 1963,• *Ketamine: a scientific review*, Celia Morgan and Valeria Curran, ISCD, September 15th 2010

48 2004 report• *Report on Ketamine*, ACMD Technical Committee, URL-21, Spring 2004

4 Why do people take drugs?

How drugs evolved

Drugs are the product of a complex evolutionary game. As fungi and plants evolved, some developed chemicals in their leaves or seeds that deterred the insects and other animals that fed on them, helping the plants to survive and reproduce. These chemicals mimicked the natural substances in insects' brains which told them how to behave, confusing the insects, or overloading their nervous systems and poisoning them.

Insects, and the larger animals that followed them, evolved in turn, adapting to these changes and sometimes developing a liking for the plant chemicals. Many animals in the wild can be seen seeking out drugs, from goats eating coffee beans, to pigs and elephants gorging on the alcohol in rotting fruit. In laboratory settings, small mammals such as mice and rats have remarkably similar reactions to humans, and become addicted to the same sort of drugs as we do. Most of the drugs we use today are either made directly from plants, or are synthetic derivatives of these plant chemicals. To understand how they work, we need to understand some of the basic mechanisms of the brain.

Chemicals in the human brain

The chemicals that send messages between nerve cells ("neurons") in our brains are called *neurotransmitters*; they respond to our environment and tell us how to behave. When we're hungry our bodies tell us to eat, and when we're full our bodies tell us to stop, just as when we're safe we need to be able to relax, and when we're in danger we need to be alert.

A neuron releases neurotransmitters into the "synapse" (gap) between this and a neighbouring neuron. The neurotransmitters move across the gap to the other neuron, where they *activate receptors* specifically designed to recognise the particular chemical (Figure 4.1), and so create feelings – for example of hunger or fear. These neurotransmitters are then reabsorbed at *reuptake sites* (Figure 4.2) when the signal isn't needed any more – for example, when a predator has gone. (At the reuptake site, special *transporter* proteins in the cell wall allow the neurotransmitter molecules, which are large, to pass into the interior of the neuron. We'll see later than some drugs work by blocking the transporters and preventing the reabsorption of the neurotransmitter.) [†]

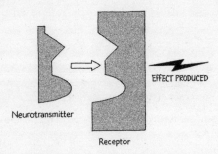

Figure 4.1: A receptor in the brain recognises a specific neurotransmitter. When the neurotransmitter activates the receptor, an effect is produced in the brain.

A typical day without drugs

The brain is extremely complex, and there's still a lot we don't know, although in the last two decades neuroimaging techniques have vastly improved our understanding of how neurotransmitters work. The most important chemicals, and a brief summary of what they do, are listed in Table 4.1 on page 54. As we'll see shortly, drugs target receptors designed to respond to these natural chemicals; the better we understand natural chemicals, the better we'll understand the effects of the drugs that mimic them.

To illustrate how these chemicals work, let's meet Ben, a clean-living man who doesn't like to take any drugs at all – not even coffee. As he

Drugs – without the hot air, David Nutt

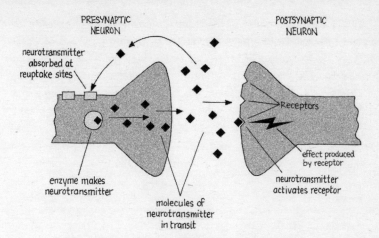

Figure 4.2: Schematic of a synapse between two neurons (nerve cells). Molecules of neurotransmitter are manufactured and emitted by the *presynaptic neuron*, and cause an effect when they activate the receptors in the *postsynaptic neuron*. The neurotransmitter can also be re-absorbed at reuptake sites, reducing the concentration of the neurotransmitter in the synapse area.

wakes up and gets out of bed, glutamate is released, kickstarting his body's transition into being awake. He drives into work, getting stuck in traffic; it's really important he's on time today, and his brain is flooded with noradrenaline as he becomes angry and stressed at the thought of being late. When he gets to work, it turns out his boss is late as well so he isn't in trouble after all, and a rise in serotonin levels makes him feel better. As lunchtime approaches, there's a dip in his cholecystokinin which makes him feel hungry, so he goes to the canteen and his cholecystokinin level rises again as he eats.

After lunch he gives an important presentation, which his boss is really pleased with, and his being congratulated causes the release of the reward chemicals endorphins and dopamine. On the way home he has an argument on the phone with his wife, and his serotonin drops making him feel miserable, but after going for a run his endorphin levels go up and he feels a lot happier. While making dinner to apologise, he cuts his finger and endocannabinoids and endorphins help numb the pain. As night falls, adenosine builds up in the brain, glutamate falls and GABA levels rise, making him feel tired and ready for sleep.

Type	Chemical	What it does
On/off switch	Glutamate	Turns the brain on: builds memory, regulates alertness, movement, sensation, and mood
On/off switch	GABA	Turns the brain off: involved in sleep, sedation, relaxation, reducing anxiety, decreasing muscle tension
Lipids	Endocannabinoids	Regulate pain, appetite, coordination, learning
Amines	Serotonin	Regulates mood and anxiety, appetite, sleep/wake cycle, body temperature
Amines	Noradrenaline (Norepinephrine in the USA)	Creates feelings of alertness, attention, concentration, raises blood pressure, lifts mood, can increase anxiety
Amines	Dopamine	Creates feelings of motivation and drive, liking, attention, pleasure, enjoyment of food
Amines	Acetylcholine	Regulates sleep/wake cycle and alertness, builds memory
Amines	Adenosine	Makes us feel tired and hungry
Peptides	Endorphins	Create feelings of pleasure and reward, reduce pain
Peptides	Substance P	Regulates pain, stress responses
Peptides	Cholecystokinin	Tells us when to eat, possibly involved in managing anxiety

Table 4.1: The brain's key communication chemicals and what they do.

What is a drug?

In the context of this book, the definition of a *drug* is a substance that comes from outside the body, crosses the blood/brain barrier, and has an effect similar to our natural neurotransmitters. (There are other types of drugs – antibiotics, asthma inhalers, warfarin, cough mixture, etc, but we're not concerned with those here.) Sometimes a drug works by blocking the reuptake sites on the synapses, so the brain experiences a surge of natural chemicals; cocaine, amphetamines and MDMA all work in this

Drugs – without the hot air, David Nutt

way. Other drugs mimic neurotransmitters (Figure 4.3), communicating with the receptors directly; alcohol and heroin both work like this, and heroin is in fact a much better fit on our endorphin receptors than the natural chemicals we produce, making it a much more effective painkiller.

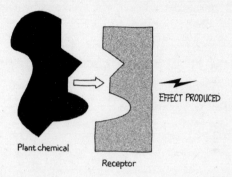

Figure 4.3: A plant chemical (a "drug") mimics the action of a normal neurotransmitter in the brain, and artificially produces an effect similar to the neurotransmitter's.

There are four main classes of drugs that are taken for pleasure, which we cover in the following sections.

1. Opioids – opium, heroin, methadone, buprenorphine, codeine

Opium, the latex of the opium poppy, has been used as a painkiller for thousands of years. It contains the opiates codeine and morphine, and from these we've also derived the synthetic opioids heroin, methadone and buprenorphine. They target the endorphin receptors in the brain, creating a dreamy sense of well-being. In medicine, they play an essential role in controlling physical pain, and are given to people with traumatic injuries or after surgery, and to enable peaceful deaths for people with terminal illnesses. They also dull psychological pain, and seem to be particularly attractive to people who've suffered psychological trauma such as child abuse or living through war.

Carrying out normal activities under the influence of opiates is pretty difficult, and even mild opiates such as codeine are not recommended for people driving or operating heavy machinery. Some are highly addictive and repeated use leads to physical dependence and powerful withdrawal symptoms. The main harms they do to the body are causing nausea, vomiting and chronic constipation, and of course the risk of death from stopping breathing in overdose.

2. Stimulants or "uppers" – cocaine, amphetamine, methamphetamine, caffeine, steroids, khat, mephedrone, tobacco

Stimulants (Table 4.2) release the amines noradrenaline and dopamine, triggering the "fight or flight" response, making you feel alert and full of energy, and suppressing the needs for food and sleep. Mild stimulants like caffeine, and nicotine (from tobacco), are part of many people's day-to-day lives, and some forms of amphetamine like Ritalin can even help people with attention disorders to concentrate on everyday tasks. Drugs at the most powerful end of the scale – cocaine, crack and methamphetamine – overstimulate the central nervous system and make focusing on normal activities difficult. The brain becomes locked onto nothing but the drug, and can't function properly.

Stimulant	Receptors targeted
cocaine	dopamine, and noradrenaline to a smaller extent
amphetamine/ methamphetamine	dopamine, and noradrenaline to a smaller extent
mephedrone	noradrenaline, dopamine, serotonin
khat	noradrenaline
caffeine	adenosine
tobacco	acetylcholine, dopamine

Table 4.2: Stimulants target a variety of receptors.

Amphetamines have a number of medicinal uses, such as treating *attention deficit hyperactivity disorder* (*ADHD*) and narcolepsy, while cocaine is a useful local anaesthetic. Soldiers, students and shift workers who need to stay alert through the night often rely on stimulants, and clubbers use them to keep dancing for hours. For people in highly-competitive environments, from street gangs to war zones to high finance, stimulants can help them cope with the psychological stress. Forms that reach the brain very quickly can be highly addictive, and regular stimulant use puts strain on the heart.

3. Depressants or "downers" – alcohol, benzodiazepines, GHB

Depressants activate the GABA receptors, so switching off the brain as though it's preparing to go to sleep. They are useful for decreasing anxiety, relieving insomnia and pain, reducing convulsions, and relaxing muscles in spasm. Alcohol is the most widely used depressant, although it also releases noradrenaline so some of its effects might appear to be like those of a stimulant. GHB is similar to alcohol. Benzodiazepines (which include Valium) are a class of medicines commonly prescribed as sleeping pills or as anxiolytics. Recreationally, all three are often combined with other drugs to counteract some of their negative effects.

Depressants seem to promote sociability and enhance mood, probably because they reduce anxiety. At low doses, or when taken as prescribed, they can be compatible with normal life – many elderly people take benzodiazepines nightly for decades to help them sleep – but higher or non-prescribed doses can lead to dependence and trouble stopping. Benzodiazepines have very few physical harms, but can impair memory and increase the risk of falls in the elderly. Alcohol is particularly damaging to the liver and brain because the body breaks alcohol down to the toxin acetaldehyde.

4. Psychedelics – LSD, mushrooms, ayuesca/DMT, peyote/mescaline, ibogaine

"Psychedelic" means "mind-manifesting", and drug of this sort are still something of a mystery to psychopharmacologists like myself. They seem to have an effect on serotonin receptors, which explains the strong pro-social feelings of openness and talkativeness they create, but it is unclear why this should be accompanied by intense visual and transcendental experiences. They very rarely produce true hallucinations (ie which have no basis in the environment), but they do produce intense visual distortions inspired by the surroundings.

Because they give insights into other ways of viewing existence, they have been used by psychotherapists to treat psychological conditions such as post-traumatic stress disorder, and to help terminal patients prepare for death. Outside of medical settings, users often take them to explore their own psychologies, and some cultures have long traditions of using them in highly-ritualised and religious settings. They are by far the least addictive class of drug, and although undertaking everyday activities is extremely difficult while under their influence, in one respect they may be easier to integrate into normal life as they rarely lead to compulsive use. They cause very little harm to the body, although nausea or vomiting are common shortly after consumption of some.

Less easily-classified drugs

Some drugs are less easy to classify. Ecstasy seems to be somewhere between a stimulant and a psychedelic, giving alertness and large amounts of energy but also producing sociability and talkativeness, because it increases serotonin by blocking serotonin reuptake. Mephedrone seems to work partly on serotonin as well. You can see how some of the most common stimulants differ from each other in terms of the neurotransmitters they target in Figure 4.4, where the higher the peak, the bigger the action of the drug.

Ketamine is another drug that falls between the classes. You could call it a depressant as it blocks glutamate, switching off the brain in a similar way that increasing GABA does (Figure 4.5), which accounts for its medicinal usefulness as an anaesthetic. Subjectively, many users liken it to a psychedelic, distorting time and space and presenting them with new perspectives.

Drugs – without the hot air, David Nutt

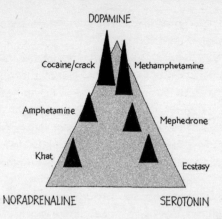

Figure 4.4: Effects of various stimulants on dopamine, noradrenaline and serotonin. The position of the peak shows the relative effect of the drug on the three different neurotransmitters. For example, khat affects noradrenaline more than dopamine or serotonin. The higher the peak, the bigger the action of the drug.

Finally, cannabis combines the feelings of relaxation typical of depressants, and distortions of perception, openness, talkativeness and great pleasure from eating. It's not surprising that cannabis has unique effects, because we have a specific natural system in the brain which the drug interacts with, known as the *endocannabinoid system*. Somewhere in our evolutionary history, cannabis must have been a very important part of the ecosystems that our animal ancestors lived in, since it developed the

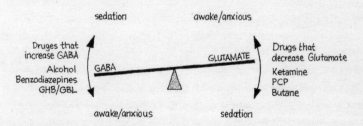

Figure 4.5: GABA and glutamate are like a see-saw, balancing sedation against anxiety/wakefulness.

ability to target one particular element of our brain chemistry so precisely!

We seem to have a particular liking for drugs that combine both sedation and stimulation. Alcohol and cannabis are the most obvious examples, but Figure 4.6 shows some others as well. One of the most popular drugs of the 20th century was Dexamyl (commonly known as Purple Hearts), an early antidepressant which appeared in the 1930s. Purple Hearts contained a combination of amphetamine (to raise mood) and barbiturates (to counteract the side-effects of the amphetamine). Even more potent were the "speedballs" invented by soldiers in Vietnam, where liquid cocaine and heroin were injected in the same syringe. It was this combination which famously killed actor River Phoenix in 1993.

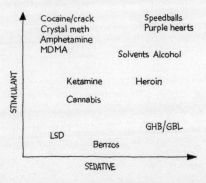

Figure 4.6: We seem to like drugs that are both stimulants and sedatives.

A typical day on drugs

Let's go back to our story about a typical day, but this time following Jen. She does all the same things as Ben, except that she, like most people, regularly uses (legal) drugs to change her brain chemistry. As she gets out of bed, her glutamate levels naturally increase, but she also drinks a cup of coffee which blocks the adenosine in her brain, making her feel more alert. When she's stressed about being stuck in traffic and her noradrenaline rises, she lights up a cigarette; the nicotine activates her

Drugs – without the hot air, David Nutt

acetylcholine receptors, calming her down. A glass of wine with lunch, (her cholecystokinin levels falling and rising again as she eats), elevates GABA, lowering her anxiety about presenting to an important client in the afternoon.

The presentation goes well, and she takes the rest of the afternoon off, supplementing the sense of well-being from dopamine and endorphins with the relaxing effects of two more glasses of wine. Her husband calls and they have an argument about whether or not she's safe to drive, which lowers her serotonin. Seeing sense, she runs home instead, stopping for a bar of chocolate which adds to the natural endorphins released by the exercise, improving her mood. She's cooking her husband a nice dinner to apologise when she cuts her finger, and doses herself with codeine to supplement her natural painkillers. Although it's been a long day, the adenosine and GABA in her brain aren't enough for her to switch off, and she lies awake for an hour before taking a Valium and falling asleep.

A brief history of drug use

Drugs can't be understood in a purely mechanical way: context and environment are essential to their effects. To understand fully their role in modern life we need to look back at the history of our interaction with them, and the steps that have brought us to this point. There have been six stages in the development of modern drugs, summarised in Figure 4.7.

The first stages were back in prehistory. Plants developed drugs to avert predators by interfering with their brains; some animals learned to overcome this aversion and to experience the chemical changes as enjoyable. Humans, with our immense curiosity, ability to remember and record experiences, and facility with tools, developed new methods for consuming drugs to deliver them to the brain more efficiently. Inhaling the smoke of the dried leaves of the tobacco plant, roasting and grinding up coffee beans, milking opium poppies for their resin and fermenting fruit and grains to make alcohol are not obvious things to do, but once

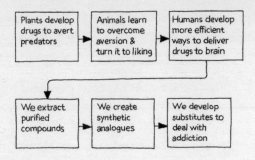

Figure 4.7: Six stages in the development of modern drugs.

we'd discovered them we found we could open up new realms of pleasurable experience. We also learned that we could heighten the effects of drugs by combining them with other substances, or encouraging the release of natural chemicals through creating euphoric or relaxing environments.

Deliberately creating altered states of consciousness is one of the human universals, like language and music. The few societies who haven't historically had some kind of botanical help have used fasting or long periods of sleeplessness to achieve these kinds of mental states, and have quickly taken to drugs like alcohol when they've encountered them. All past societies used plants and herbs as medicines, and were aware of the importance of dosage – that even the most beneficial or pleasurable drug could become a poison at a higher enough dose.

Although changing our consciousness with drugs has been common to almost all societies, for most of human history the plants and substances available were limited to what grew nearby, and what each culture had come to understand as enjoyable. As a result, the drugs that were known and used in different parts of the world were relatively static.

It's hard to know exactly when different drugs came into use, but a thousand years ago a traveller would probably have encountered a world like that shown in Figure 4.8. The traveller would have found that each of the drugs shown had a specific cultural context, and was loaded with social, religious and political meanings. The psychedelics peyote, ayuesca,

Drugs – without the hot air, David Nutt

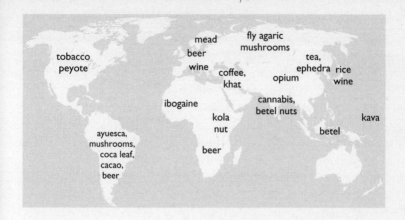

Figure 4.8: A map of the world showing the main drugs in use 1000 years ago.

ibogaine and fly agaric mushrooms were an essential part of religious rituals and shamanic trances, just as wine had a prescribed role in many Jewish rituals. Switching from one intoxicant to another sometimes accompanied major cultural changes, such as the replacement of alcohol with coffee in the Arab world with the rise of Islam. Kava drinking in the Pacific and smoking tobacco in peace pipes in the Americas played important roles in maintaining social cohesion, while also cementing gender divides, as women weren't allowed to consume them. Sometimes substances that we would consider drugs today were seen as food, and vice versa: beer played an essential role in the diets of northern Europe in the past, because water was usually contaminated with bacteria. In Latin America, cacao was treated as a kind of medicine when Western explorers first encountered it.

As travel became easier and more common, medications and pleasure drugs were introduced to new places. The empires that emerged in places like China and the Middle East spread knowledge about the natural world, and most of the standard therapies available in medieval England were derived from Greek or Islamic sources. European expansion spread drugs and medicines as well as disease. Explorers brought back tobacco and cacao (and probably syphilis too) from the Americas, and coffee was adopted in Europe with the expansion of the Ottoman Empire. Over the course of a few centuries, the drugs available in many parts of the world multiplied, creating new social contexts.

It was advances in chemistry, however, which created recognisably modern drugs. In 1817, a young German called Friedrich Sertürner was the first to isolate in its pure form the active ingredient from a plant, extracting morphine from opium. That made it possible to study pure psychoactive compounds, and develop medicines that were far stronger and more effective than the plants they were derived from. Once we understood the make up of these chemicals, we could produce them synthetically in the laboratory, and it was only a short step from there to experimenting with the psychoactive effects of chemically similar compounds. Heroin, amphetamines and mephedrone are, respectively, synthetic analogues of the opium found in poppies, the ephedra found in ephedra plants, and the cathinone found in khat.

This revolutionised medicine, but also led to huge problems. Before the 19th century, the majority of medicines that ordinary people had access to were probably inert, having very little effect at all. By the late 1800s, pretty much everything on sale in the pharmacy, including cough medicines for children, contained extracts of cannabis, heroin or cocaine. The lack of regulation about what medicines contained, who could get hold of them and what the appropriate dosage might be, had allowed medicinal companies to generate profits while putting many people at risk of dependence and overdose. This led to many governments bringing in strict regulation about labelling and distribution, and eventually to international treaties that made these substances illegal.

These new drugs were powerful and immensely pleasurable, and humans are programmed to want to repeat pleasurable experiences. We'll look at the concept of addiction in detail in chapter 8, but its defining feature is that the user has such powerful cravings for the drug that they find it almost impossible to resist taking it, even if it is destroying their relationships, their health, or their ability to lead a normal life. Unfortunately, as we've developed more and more efficient ways of delivering drugs to the brain we've inevitably made them more and more

Drugs – without the hot air, David Nutt

addictive. These leaps forward in medicine and our understanding of the brain have had unintended consequences, and pharmacologists now spend a lot of time researching substitutes for common drugs of abuse, in the hope of finding less harmful ones.

Why do people take drugs?

Let's go back to the opening question: why do people take drugs? Looking at how drugs came to exist, it would be surprising if we *didn't* take them. Plants were producing chemicals especially designed to interfere with animals' brains long before humans existed, and humans have evolved to respond to their effects just as we've evolved to digest certain foods. Cultures that haven't employed the psychoactive powers of plants have been in the minority, and have used other methods to alter their states of consciousness. From this point of view, taking drugs is entirely natural; as Mike Jay puts it in his book †*High Society*, "we were taking drugs long before we were human".

We use drugs for two main reasons: to experience pleasure, and to relieve suffering. These could crudely be referred to as "recreational" and "medicinal" drug use, but although the †international treaties of the 1960s created a strict legal division between the two, in reality the line between them is very blurred. The most obvious examples are drugs such as cannabis and LSD which are placed in Schedule I (with no recognised medicinal value), so that any use at all is seen as "recreational", despite the fact that many people with conditions like multiple sclerosis (MS) or cluster headaches are demonstrably reducing their suffering by taking them. Other drugs which have recognised but limited medicinal uses, such as heroin for extreme pain, may still be reducing suffering when taken outside of an obviously therapeutic context. For people who have experienced serious trauma (such as soldiers with PTSD) taking a drug like heroin might be the only thing that makes their lives liveable. Alcohol is often used to self-medicate, as we discuss below.

The use of drugs for pleasure has a number of elements beyond their mechanical effects on our brains. Indeed, we have to be *expecting* to experience pleasure: most of us would find taking a drug by accident deeply unpleasant, and would think that we had been poisoned or were having a psychotic episode. Actively choosing to take a drug is an essential part of the effect it has, and even animals experience different effects depending on whether or not they've chosen to consume it. †Rats that are passively given cocaine injections will become physically dependent on the drug (experiencing withdrawal symptoms if they stop), but become much more addicted – in terms of actively seeking out the drug – when they have to push a lever themselves to self-administer it.

Drugs are social, and are usually consumed in groups, where the feelings of disinhibition and talkativeness that many drugs generate help promote social bonding. Using a particular substance, or using it in a particular way, can become a strong marker of identity, and can herald important social changes. †Coca chewing has become more popular in Bolivia since the election of an indigenous president, for example, and †greater gender equality has often been accompanied by increased rates of smoking amongst women. Refusing to participate in drug-taking can feel very uncomfortable, as teenagers know when they struggle with peer pressure, and as many adults experience if we refuse the offer of an alcoholic drink in the pub.

The use of some drugs, especially psychedelics, can be heavily imbued with meaning. Taking psychoactive substances in religious settings and rituals is called *entheogenic* drug use, and blurs the line between what is recreational and medicinal. Sometimes these occasions are explicitly for healing purposes, although it may be the shaman who takes the drug rather than the patient. (This was how tobacco was used in some traditional Native American ceremonies.) In other cases, the drug is used to access secret knowledge or divine experience. It may be only the shaman who consumes the drug, or it may be the entire congregation, as with †the Native American Church's use of peyote. While entheogenic drug use may have pleasurable moments of euphoria and ecstasy, these experiences are often described as painfully intense, an ordeal to be struggled through rather than an escapist "trip". This makes them very different

Drugs – without the hot air, David Nutt

from, for example, the use of LSD in a dance club setting, as was recognised in 1996 when the Native American Church was granted special dispensation to use peyote in their services.

Sometimes people get pleasure from taking drugs precisely because it is risky. This is particularly noticeable when prescribed medicines get diverted: †American schoolchildren who take Ritalin illicitly have quite different reactions to those who take it as directed by their doctor. (An illicit activity is illegal in one context but might be legal under other circumstances – for example, if your grandmother has a prescription for Valium she can take it legally, but if you take her Valium that's illegal/illicit drug use.) In recent years, a new trend has emerged amongst young people in the UK, of deliberately trying to get so intoxicated (usually on alcohol) that they have no memory of getting "wasted" or "ended". It can be hard to understand why this would be pleasurable, but it probably relates to the social kudos of the things people feel permitted to do while extremely disinhibited.

The use of alcohol in British society today illustrates how difficult it can be to separate the use of drugs to relieve suffering from their use for pleasure. At the most extreme end, people with low levels of GABA receptors who live in a chronic state of anxiety may feel "normal" only when they drink. While it's certainly not the ideal medication, their drinking isn't primarily motivated by pleasure. At the less severe end of the scale, there are millions of people in the UK who find it very difficult to wind down after work without alcohol – a sort of mild self-medication against the stress of their working lives. Of course, this often takes place in the pub, and chatting to friends and relaxing is pleasurable as well as medicinal. The drug, combined with the sociable context of the pub, makes people feel both "better" and "good", and if this is where most of their social life takes place, not going to the pub in order to cut down on their alcohol intake will make them feel miserable and isolated.

Finally, a minority of drug users will take them because they are addicted, which we'll explore in greater detail in chapter 8. Addiction blurs the line between pain and pleasure. It is quite common for someone to start taking a drug for the enjoyable effects, but once they're addicted it becomes the only thing that can relieve the intense cravings and unpleasant physical symptoms of withdrawal.

Why this matters

Humans have always deliberately consumed psychoactive substances, and our brains are adapted to respond to them. However, although in this sense drug-taking is "natural", the purified drugs we now have access to, and the speed with which we can get them into the brain, make many of them far more potent than the drugs we evolved with. This makes them more effective and potentially more harmful. We need to understand both our natural impulses and the contemporary cultural context of drug-taking if we want to reduce these harms.

In medicine, the idea that we're always weighing up the costs of a drug against its benefits is well understood, if not always perfectly enacted. With some drugs, the benefits are not officially recognised; with others, it's not clear if it's the patient, the doctor, the regulatory body or pharmaceutical company that should ultimately decide if the cost/benefit ratio of a drug is worthwhile. But at least harm minimisation is understood to involve the balancing of two risks (the risk of remaining ill, and the risk of being harmed by the drug), rather than seeing the drug solely as a source of harm. No government would make it their policy to reduce the number of people taking medications if these medications were improving the health of the nation overall.

When it comes to minimising the harms of recreational drug use, there are several schools of thought. One aims to eradicate the decadent use of drugs altogether – the "drug-free world" that the 1961 UN Single Convention on Drugs aimed to create. This plays well in the tabloids, but is very flawed in practice. For a start, there are measurable benefits to a life which includes pleasure, so eradicating pleasurable drug use could cause other sorts of harm, such as an increase in stress-related health problems. This is understood with alcohol, and sociable drinking or drinking to unwind after work is genuinely beneficial (although the harms are also very real). The government can certainly make it easier for people to enjoy the benefits of the pub while doing themselves less damage, by making alcohol more expensive, ensuring that non-alcoholic drinks are cheaper and more widely available, or funding research into a safer alternative. But banning pubs altogether would damage people's health in other ways, as well as causing public outrage.

There is also an entirely practical reason for accepting that a level of excessive drug use is always going to be part of human society: we simply don't know how to stop it. Humans are natural pleasure seekers. As part of our brain's normal functioning, it releases endorphins and dopamine to generate feelings of wellbeing from doing a job well, spending time with people we love, meditation, prayer, and collective activities like singing and dancing. These feelings of well-being create memories which teach us which experiences we should repeat. Drugs interact with these natural learning systems in a very powerful way, often creating some of the most intense experiences a person ever has. We are programmed to enjoy these experiences, and even very severe punishment doesn't necessarily act as a deterrent, though it will create all sorts of other kinds of harm.

If we accept that people are going to take drugs for pleasure, and that the important thing is to minimise harm, then understanding the reasons behind drug use can give us inspiration as to how this should be achieved. If part of the pleasure of the drug is the positive social context it is consumed in, then it might be possible to create similar contexts where the drug is not the focus, such as the measures proposed above to make the pub less harmful. On the other hand, if people are specifically looking for a risky experience, they are going to expose themselves to harm whatever drugs they take. Challenging the culture of extreme intoxication is one of the most difficult tasks we face, but it is essential if harm is going to be reduced. One of the best protections against this kind of risk-taking is allowing positive cultures to develop around drugs that emphasise moderate consumption rather than bingeing – in a sense, creating entheogenic-type social contexts similar to traditional uses of psychedelics and other substances. This would help protect against the acute problems of extreme intoxication, and also against addiction: [†]Native Americans avoided becoming addicted to tobacco for thousands of years by surrounding its use with ritual and having strictly-observed restrictions on when and how it was taken. While this kind of context is unlikely to develop in the UK, a renewed sense of a social code of acceptable and unacceptable behaviour when taking drugs like alcohol and cocaine would certainly help to reduce harm.

Drugs are an important part of our evolutionary history, and we are surrounded by them every day. Most of us take drugs of some form on a daily basis, and appreciate the benefits they bring. Becoming more aware of the reasons we like them so much, and how we can maximise their beneficial aspects while minimising the harm they do, is a challenge that needs to be taken up by individuals, communities and governments.

Notes

Page

52 •Recommended reading on neurotransmitters: *The Atlas of Psychiatric Pharmacotherapy*, Roni Shiloh and David Nutt et al, Taylor & Francis, 2006

65 *High Society*, "we were taking drugs long before we were human"• *High Society*, Mike Jay, Thames & Hudson, 2010

65 international treaties of the 1960s created a strict legal division between the two• *Single Convention on Narcotic Drugs*, UN, URL-22, 1961 (amended 1972)

66 Rats that are passively given cocaine injections• *Differences in extracellular dopamine concentrations in the nucleus accumbens during response-dependent and response-independent cocaine administration in the rat*, SE Hemby et al, Psychopharmacology (Berlin) 133(1), September 1997

66 Coca chewing has become more popular in Bolivia since the election of an indigenous president• *The Wonders of the Coca Leaf*, Alan Forsberg, URL-23, 2007

66 greater gender equality has often been accompanied by increased rates of smoking amongst women• *Gender empowerment and female-to-male smoking prevalence ratios*, Sara Hitchman and Geoffrey Fong, Bulletin of the World Health Organization, URL-24, January 5th 2011

66 the Native American Church's use of peyote• *American Indian Religious Freedom Act*, URL-25, 1996

67 American schoolchildren who take Ritalin illicitly have quite different reactions to those who take it as directed by their doctor.• *Evidence-based guidelines for management of attention-deficit/hyperactivity disorder in adolescents in transition to adult services and in adults: recommendations from the British Association for Psychopharmacology*, David Nutt et al, Journal of Psychopharmacology (21), 2006

70 Native Americans avoided becoming addicted to tobacco for thousands of years• *Tobacco use by Native Americans: sacred smoke and silent killer*, Joseph Winter (ed.), University of Oklahoma Press, 2000

5 Cannabis, and why did Queen Victoria take it?

The cannabis plant originated in Asia and has been used by humans for thousands of years. The plant has had three lives: as a fibre, as a medicine, and as a pleasure drug. In its first life we have hemp, one of the most versatile plant fibres in nature; in the second we have cannabis indica, which relieves pain and spasm; and in its third we have "ganja", "weed" or "skunk", the most widely-used recreational drug in the world today after alcohol and tobacco. Over the last century, these three lives have interwoven, creating a complicated legal situation which causes a great deal of harm to many millions around the globe. This chapter looks at the benefits and harms of the drug, and tells the story of how the world's oldest medicine lost its therapeutic value on the international stage.

Cannabis as hemp

The stem of the cannabis plant can be used to make hemp, which was an essential commodity for making ropes in seafaring societies such as the ancient Greeks and the British in times past. †Henry VIII even passed a law requiring farmers to grow it! Nowadays, hemp is used for special paper, such as for banknotes and bibles, for fabrics, and for a low-carbon building material called "hempcrete", which is a mixture of hemp and lime. The varieties grown for these purposes have only trace psychoactive properties.

Cannabis as a drug

The psychoactive parts of cannabis are the buds and resin of the female plants, which can be eaten, smoked in a water pipe or combined with tobacco in a cigarette, known as a "spliff" or "joint". The resin is generally known as "hash" and the buds as "weed", and the whole plant is also known by its Mexican name marihuana or marijuana. A more potent form of weed known as "skunk" has appeared in the last decade, the product of plants specially bred in European laboratories.

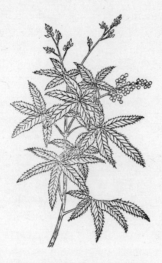

Figure 5.1: The cannabis plant.

The psychoactive ingredient in cannabis is *tetrahydrocannabinol* (*THC*), [†]and the receptors it acts on are named *cannabis receptors*. When scientists began looking for the naturally-occurring neurotransmitters that these must have evolved to recognise, they found a control system that helps regulate appetite, pain sensation, mood and memory. This is known as the *endocannabinoid system*, and the naturally-occurring chemicals that activate it were named *endocannabinoids*, from "endogenous cannabinoids".

Cannabis usually makes users feel relaxed, talkative and sociable – known colloquially as being "stoned". It can produce a distorted sense of time and space, although not as severely as psychedelic drugs. Some people can also experience paranoia. Although by no means safe, it is considerably less harmful than alcohol, and rarely induces violence or antisocial behaviour.

What are the benefits?

Cannabis is probably the world's oldest medicine, used mainly for treating pain and spasm. It's known as [†]"ma" in Chinese medicine, a pun on the word "chaotic", and was historically used largely in a therapeutic context, although a minority also used it as an intoxicant. While medical uses have long been known in Indian medicine as well, where it's known as [†]"bhang", there is also a long history of widespread use for recreational purposes, and the plant and its psychoactive properties are a common feature in Indian legends and folktales. Even today it is used in certain festivals.

Although cannabis was known to Western medicine in the middle ages, [†]it was only popularised in Britain in the 1840s, by an army surgeon who had served in India. Cannabis became a common painkiller, alongside opium (laudanum). It is thought that Queen Victoria's physician JR Reynolds prescribed it to help her with period pains and after childbirth. In the *Lancet*, Reynolds wrote a paper entitled *On the Therapeutic Uses and Toxic Effects of Cannabis Indica*, in which he said [†]"when pure and administered carefully, it is one of the most valuable medicines we possess". Queen Victoria was apparently very fond of it – perhaps getting access to cannabis was one of the reasons she had so many children!

[†]The condition that seems to benefit most commonly from the use of cannabis is multiple sclerosis (MS), a disease characterised by fatigue, muscle weakness, incontinence, muscle spasms and chronic pain. About 85,000 people in the UK suffer from MS, and at least 1% of these self-medicate with cannabis. Sufferers say that the drug helps with spasticity, pain, tremor and urinary bladder control, and even though the drug is illegal many doctors do not discourage their patients from self-administering it.

Drugs – without the hot air, David Nutt

†Cannabis also seems to have benefits in a number of other disorders, such as relieving the pain from a phantom limb among amputees, and preventing seizures in epileptics. There is anecdotal evidence that it may be useful in treating glaucoma and bronchial asthma, as it lowers the pressure in the eye and dilates the small airways of the lung.

Other therapeutic uses of cannabis include helping underweight people, such as those with cancer and AIDS, bulk up by increasing their appetite – wanting to eat after taking cannabis is a common effect of the drug, known colloquially as "the munchies". And although cannabis can worsen psychotic symptoms, it does seem to have some antipsychotic effects as well, which may account for its popularity with people suffering from schizophrenia. (See box *Does cannabis cause schizophrenia?* on page 85.)

Recreationally, cannabis serves a similar role to alcohol as a social lubricant, particularly as there is a long established culture of sharing the drug – it's extremely rude not to pass the spliff! It is also popular with artists and musicians, and there are †many accounts of its helping inspire people's creativity. Some say that the whole genre of jazz emerged as cannabis allowed musicians to break free of conventional music structure and syncopate!

What are the harms?

While cannabis is considerably less damaging than alcohol, it still †scored 20 on our harm scale. This might surprise some people, particularly those who are experienced with the drug and view it as harmless. Over the 16 criteria, it scored highest on drug-related damage and drug-related impairment of mental functioning, mostly because of the harms associated with smoking, and the drug's links with depression and psychotic symptoms.

†Cannabis dependence occurs in about 10% of users, and there is a physical withdrawal syndrome with some unpleasant symptoms, such as decreased appetite, weight loss, mood changes and insomnia. These are real and not just psychosomatic: drugs like †rimonabant, which

block the effects of cannabis, can precipitate these withdrawal symptoms. (This distinction is explained more fully in chapter 8.) Even without physical symptoms, many regular users experience psychological craving if they stop. [†]In the UK in 2007/8, around 17,000 people were treated for cannabis addiction, half of them under 18, and the problem is probably much more widespread.

Often the biggest effect that cannabis has on people's lives is a general sense of demotivation and lack of enjoyment of activities when not intoxicated, and if used regularly, especially daily, it can disrupt school work or employment. [†]A study of US postal workers found lower levels of attainment among people who tested positive for cannabis, and research has shown that long-term use can affect cognitive skills, making it harder to learn and retain information.

Being illegal, there are other harms associated with the production and distribution of cannabis. Most of the drug used in the UK is now sourced domestically, often being grown on farms run by criminal gangs who channel the proceeds into other sorts of crime, such as people trafficking. In recent years, many of the farms have started being run by [†]Vietnamese gangs, who use illegal Vietnamese immigrants (some of them children) as workers in conditions of near-slave labour.

Cannabis routes of use

There are three traditional methods ("routes of use") of taking cannabis, and a fourth for Sativex, a medicinally approved cannabis spray. In increasing order of harmfulness, they are:

1. Spraying the medicinal form on the back of your throat. The spray is the least harmful route, as you would expect with a medically approved substance.
2. Eating (usually cooked in sweet foods like cookies) is probably the second least harmful as it also avoids the health problems associated with smoking, but it can take up to 4 hours to reach the brain (Figure 5.2), and this delayed effect does make it harder to judge the dose.

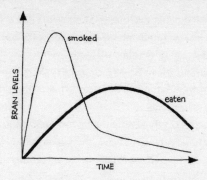

Figure 5.2: Because cannabis reaches the brain more slowly when eaten than when smoked, judging the dose when it is eaten is more difficult.

3. Inhaling through a water pipe known as a bong is intuitively cleaner than smoking, but because people don't choke or cough they can take much deeper breaths and get more intoxicated. A subculture of rapid bong inhalation to extreme levels of intoxication has emerged, which seems to be different in character to the "chilled out" attitude of people who prefer spliffs.

4. Smoking cannabis with tobacco in cigarettes puts the smokers at risk of the same problems that smoking tobacco alone does;

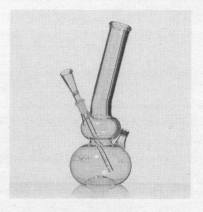

Figure 5.3: A bong.

smoking cannabis pure reduces these risks, but it doesn't remove them completely. Spliffs are usually passed around a group rather than smoked by an individual, but users usually inhale more deeply than they do with tobacco alone, and often hold the smoke for 10–15 seconds as they believe this makes them more "stoned". (†Tests have shown that this doesn't actually increase THC levels in the brain, so it is probably just oxygen deprivation that causes the bigger effect.)

Is skunk more harmful than hash?

In the 1990s, much of the cannabis consumed in the UK was hash imported from Morocco, but as the War on Drugs started to clamp down on production there, Moroccan hash became more difficult to get hold of. In response, criminal gangs in northern Europe started to grow their own, and selectively bred cannabis plants to increase the THC levels, creating new breeds generally known as skunk because of their powerful unpleasant smell. Most skunk has about two or three times the THC content of unmodified weed or hash.

Skunk is potentially more harmful than hash because it contains less *cannabidiol* (*CBD*), a psychoactive compound that reduces anxiety and can minimise some of the negative effects of THC. Breeding more THC into skunk has resulted in CBD being bred out. However, we don't know whether people using skunk actually take in more THC, because there's some evidence that experienced users vary how deeply they breathe to keep an even level of THC intoxication; this is called "titrating the dose". Other research has found that products with higher THC levels are less well liked – tests on hash smokers have found that they find skunk too strong, and that many people would rather smoke hash if they could get hold of it. This seems to have been recognised by cannabis producers, and although †THC levels were at one point as high as 21%, they soon dropped back down to 15%, which was clearly a more pleasurable and saleable strength.

Drugs – without the hot air, David Nutt

Why did cannabis stop being seen as a medicine?

The story of how cannabis became a much-feared recreational drug and lost its status as a medicine is rather complicated. Cannabis was used in Asia both medicinally and recreationally for many thousands of years, while the plant was ubiquitous across Europe as the source of hemp, from at least the Middle Ages. However, there seems to have been very little recreational use of the plant in Europe, partly because these varieties were low in THC, and partly because smoking was essentially unknown in Europe until Christopher Columbus came across Native Americans smoking tobacco. Even when pipe-smoking of tobacco became more common, and cannabis started being used as a medicine, there was almost no recreational use of the drug in Britain until the late 19th century, and levels remained very low until the 1960s.

Of course, the British government did encounter widespread use of the drug as the British Empire expanded into Asia. Here it was viewed as a commodity, which, because it was seen as an essential daily item by many Indians, could be used as a means of social control. Just as the East India company cornered the market in salt, they shut down the local production of cannabis, forcing people to buy their "bhang" from the British. (When you factor-in the opium trade in China, and the vast profits made from trading tea, coffee and alcohol, the British Empire was easily the largest drug dealer in the history of the world!)

When cannabis entered the physician's medicine chest in Britain in the 1840s, it was †overshadowed by the more potent painkilling properties of opium, partly because opium was easier to convert into other forms such as laudanum, morphine and heroin. Cannabis tinctures (extract dissolved in alcohol) were sold as cures for cramp, opiate withdrawal, migraines and insomnia, and enjoyed a brief period of popularity in Britain towards the end of the century. However, growing concern about unregulated medicines led to the British Medical Association launching its campaign against "Secret Remedies" in the early 1900s, after which cannabis was removed from most of these medications, as were cocaine, morphine and heroin.

Meanwhile, some British governors in India were becoming worried that cannabis might be causing widespread psychological problems in the colony. This led to the †Indian Hemp Drugs Commission report in 1894, which assembled seven volumes' worth of evidence on the medicinal and social uses of cannabis in the subcontinent. The report concluded that the drug was not harmful, and should not be controlled. Yet the report was largely ignored in the UK, despite having been commissioned by the British Parliament and having collected a huge variety of testimony and evidence, and it was not even mentioned in Parliament until 1967. The legal status of cannabis, and its possible harms and benefits, were seen as a foreign issue unrelated to everyday British concerns.

This lack of interest shaped Britain's response at the international level. In 1925 Egypt, backed by Turkey, proposed that cannabis be included in the Geneva International Convention on Narcotics Control. This was ostensibly on the grounds that "chronic hashism" was causing widespread insanity, although since this wasn't occurring in India (and still doesn't in present-day Britain, for that matter), this was almost certainly an exaggeration of the problem. Egypt did, however, rely heavily on cotton exports, and may have been trying to protect its cotton industry from the competition posed by hemp cloth. The vote went in Egypt's favour, despite opposition from India, and although the British delegate made a show of support for the colony by abstaining from the vote, Britain still signed the treaty.

The 1925 treaty led to the Dangerous Drugs Act in the UK, which came into force in 1928, banning the recreational use of opium, cannabis and cocaine. (Opium and cocaine had already been controlled for a decade by the 1916 Defence of the Realm Act.) All three drugs were still available as medicines, and recreational use was rare, so this passed without much comment. While the media featured occasional stories about "dope fiends" – foreign men using drugs to corrupt white women – there was nowhere near the same level of hysteria in Britain as in the USA (described below), and cannabis was rarely mentioned in these tales. †In 1945 there were a total of 4 prosecutions for cannabis offences, and it wasn't until 1950 that the number of prosecutions for cannabis (86)

Drugs – without the hot air, David Nutt

outnumbered those for opium and other manufactured drugs (83). There was no domestic pressure to control cannabis alongside other hard drugs – and equally, no organised effort to keep it legal.

†The situation was very different in the USA. The Geneva International Convention was convened by the League of Nations, which the USA never joined, so cannabis in the USA was controlled later than elsewhere, with the Marijuana Tax of 1937. This prohibited the sale or growth of cannabis without a tax stamp which, although it only cost one dollar, was never made publicly available, effectively outlawing production. This was the culmination of several decades of increasing concern about the drug's recreational uses, fuelled by exaggerated reports in the media about its harmful effects.

In the USA, cannabis was strongly associated with immigrants from Mexico, and even the spelling was altered from "marihuana" to "marijuana" (to rhyme with Tijuana) to make it seem more Mexican. Among the most vocal part of the press spreading rumours about its negative effects were the outlets owned by William Randolph Hearst, a media tycoon who had invested heavily in the wood pulp industry. Since hemp paper posed direct competition to wood pulp paper, he had an economic stake in limiting hemp production, and recognised that if controls were placed on cannabis because of its psychoactive effects, it would become more difficult to grow the plant for other purposes. Hearst's media empire spread stories about violent attacks on white women by Mexican immigrants intoxicated with marijuana, creating a sense of moral panic and support for controls on the drug, and therefore on the plant as well.

The three lives of cannabis now became dependent on the fate of its use as a recreational drug. Although ordinary Americans were familiar with hemp, many didn't realise that it had anything to do with marijuana, just as many doctors didn't realise it was the same plant as *cannabis indica*, which they considered a valuable medicine. By the time the USA was leading the negotiations behind the 1961 UN Single Convention on Drugs, the view of cannabis was so dim that, not only was it placed in the same category of harmfulness as cocaine and opiates, but whereas those drugs were still allowed some medical use, WHO (the World Health

Organization) declared that cannabis had no medical value at all.

This anomaly may have been partly due to the complexity of cannabis as a compound. Whereas opium and cocaine were strongly promoted by the pharmaceutical industry, cannabis had fallen out of favour with drug companies when they started extracting pure ingredients from various drugs to produce medicines in pill form, and when the hypodermic syringe was invented. Cannabis doesn't dissolve in water so it can't be injected, and it is too complex to make into tablets (in the same way that you can't make tablets out of tobacco). This lack of support from pharmaceutical companies, combined with hostility from industries in competition with hemp, and outrage at the supposed violence and insanity that cannabis could cause, led to it being devalued as a medicine.

In Britain, cannabis continued to be available on prescription throughout the 1960s. However, this was the decade in which recreational use became common, with some people buying it on the black market, and others [†]diverting prescriptions from their doctors. Although cannabis users and medical professionals had become more organised by this point, and were trying to get the drug decriminalised for all uses, some of the moral panic from the USA had been imported, and there was a lot of political pressure to control the drug still further. After the 1971 UN Convention on Psychotropic Substances, the British government decided [†]not to renew the medical licence on cannabis, in part because of concerns about the drug being diverted from medical sources. This was an odd way to have dealt with the problem. Doctors have access to a wide range of other drugs with abuse potential, and we stop those supplies being diverted by having strict rules and regulations around what doctors can prescribe, and by disciplining them through the General Medical Council if they break those rules. It was the doctors' practice that needed to be banned, not the drug.

Medicinal cannabis use in the UK today

The criminalisation of cannabis (Figure 5.4) for recreational use has resulted in a great deal of harm from imprisonment, as we'll discuss in

Drugs – without the hot air, David Nutt

chapter 15. However, the most inhumane result of the legal status of cannabis has been the criminalisation of very sick and disabled people who rely on the drug as a medicine. A middle-aged ex-teacher with MS wrote to me recently detailing how the police have broken down her front door in dawn raids on three occasions in the last six years to combat her use of cannabis for medical purposes. This kind of aggressive law enforcement is devastating for the patients and their families and distasteful for the courts – many magistrates will privately admit their extreme dislike of having to criminalise users. And that's not to mention its being a complete waste of public money.

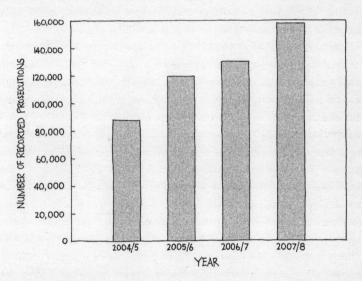

Figure 5.4: Number of recorded cannabis possession offences. (Source: Crime Statistics, Home Office.)

In 1998, [†]the House of Lords Select Committee produced a report into the medical uses of cannabis and the effects of criminalisation on its users. They recommended that all criminal sanctions against such users be dropped, and that a cannabis-based medicine should be approved for prescription within three years. In fact, it took until 2010 for the cannabis spray Sativex to receive approval in Britain; even this doesn't meet the needs of all patients, and is available only if the doctor is willing to prescribe it, which most still aren't. If anything, †the legal situation has become even more draconian in recent years. In 2005, the Court of Appeal ruled that the Defence of Necessity was no longer admissible in cases where patients have been found growing or possessing cannabis to treat a medical problem for which other treatments were ineffective.

Those forced to plead guilty to possession of a Class B drug rarely face prison, but can receive substantial fines and suffer a great deal of mental distress, anxiety and social humiliation. Some have also had their possessions and bank accounts seized under the new Proceeds of Crime legislation, where there is evidence that the offender has "benefited" from his or her "criminal conduct".

This terribly unjust situation surely cannot be allowed continue, especially once Sativex has been rescheduled to make the law consistent. At the time of writing, the medicine has been approved under a general licence, avoiding the fact that the drug it contains is in Schedule 1, with no recognised medical use. The ACMD has recommended that Sativex be rescheduled to Schedule 4, along with other medicines such as benzodiazepines and anabolic steroids. However, any such legislation will have to name the active components rather than use the trade name Sativex. It has been suggested that it be described as an extract of THC and CBD, but this is inadequate as Sativex also contains dozens of other cannabinoids which occur naturally in the plant. It is very hard to get around the fact that the only accurate description for the medicine is "cannabis". This will be quite a conundrum for politicians such as Minister for Crime Prevention †James Brokenshire, who has insisted in Parliament that cannabis in its "raw form" is a harmful drug with no medical purposes, and then asserted in the same breath that Sativex is a "safe and effective" treatment for MS.

Conclusion

The three stories of the cannabis plant – as pleasure drug, medicine and plant fibre – show that many different factors have contributed to the

Drugs – without the hot air, David Nutt

legal situation we have today. Rather than being based on a rational assessment of the harms and benefits of the drug, the current legal status of cannabis in the UK is the result of factors such as Egyptian domestic politics in the 1920s, a handful of British doctors misprescribing medicinal cannabis in the 1960s, and industrial interests in the USA who wanted to stop hemp production. To this day, [†]no varieties of hemp can be grown in the US, not even the versions that are used in Europe, which have no psychoactive properties.

The negative effects of this situation are felt far and wide. A lot of young people ignore the genuine warnings that health professionals give them about the dangers of cannabis, because so many of these warnings are exaggerated. Rather than protecting people, exaggerated warnings increase the risks of harm and addiction. Criminalising recreational use leads to thousands of young people getting a criminal record each year for using a drug which is considerably less harmful than alcohol. While these consequences cause a lot of suffering, the negative effects of criminalising the *medicinal* use of cannabis are even worse. As a result of laws which had almost nothing to do with the risks or benefits of the drug, thousands of sick and disabled people are denied access to a medicine with unique properties for treating their illnesses, or are forced to break the law and risk prosecution to obtain it. This nonsensical and inhumane situation cannot continue, and our trust in politicians is eroded when they make statements that draw a false distinction between "raw cannabis" and the cannabis-based medicines they have licensed. We must base our laws on a realistic assessment of harm, not on irrelevant historical factors, nor on political cowardice about changing the status quo.

Does cannabis cause schizophrenia?

In 2007, the Home Secretary [†]requested the ACMD to review the status of cannabis for the third time in six years because [†]"Though statistics show that cannabis use has fallen significantly, there is real public concern about the potential mental-health effects of cannabis use, in particular the use of stronger forms of the drug, commonly known as skunk." The ACMD's resulting report looked at this question in depth.

There has been a lot of commentary and some research as to whether cannabis is associated with schizophrenia, and the results are really quite difficult to interpret. What we can say is that cannabis use is associated with an increased incidence of psychotic disorders, particularly short-term episodes. Analysing this is complicated because the reason people take cannabis is precisely because it produces a change in their mental state. These changes are the nearest that most people get to experiencing what it is like to be psychotic – they include distortions of perception (especially in visual and auditory perception) as well as in the way one thinks. So it can be quite hard to know whether, when you analyse the incidence of psychotic disorders with cannabis, you are simply looking at the acute (ie short-term) effects of cannabis, as opposed to some more enduring consequence of cannabis use.

There are many other confounding factors that make it hard to prove that a specific patient's schizophrenia has been caused by cannabis. Schizophrenia usually develops in the late teens and early 20s, which is also the age group that uses the most cannabis. Schizophrenia is more common among those with low socio-economic status and those who have experienced childhood trauma, both of which are associated with higher levels of drug use and addiction. Cannabis does seem to relieve some of the symptoms of schizophrenia, even though it sometimes worsens others, so there could be an element of reverse causality – the psychosis may lead to cannabis use, not the other way round. And it's very possible that there is a gene that predisposes people to both schizophrenia and liking cannabis, neither really causing the other.

If we err on the cautious side, we can say that if you take cannabis, particularly if you use a lot of it, you will be more likely to have psychotic experiences. That includes schizophrenia, but the rarity of the condition, and the confounding factors discussed above, make it very hard to be sure about its causation. The analysis we came up with was that smokers of cannabis are about 2.6 times more likely to have a psychotic-like experience than non-smokers. To put that figure in proportion, you are 20 times more likely to get lung cancer if you smoke tobacco than if you don't: there is a relatively small risk that smoking cannabis will lead to psychotic illness compared with quite a substantial risk for smoking tobacco and developing lung cancer.

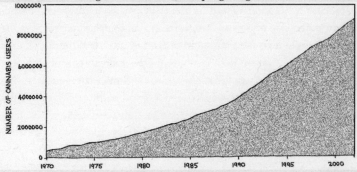

Figure 5.5: Use of cannabis in England and Wales, 1970–2002. Source OCJS Survey.

Another confounding factor is that schizophrenia seems to be reducing in the general population even though cannabis use has increased 20-fold in the last 40 years ([†]Figure 5.5). Figures from the General Practice Research Database in the UK consistently and clearly [†]show that psychosis and schizophrenia are still on the decline. So, even though skunk has been around now for ten years, there has been no upswing in schizophrenia. In fact, where people have looked, they haven't found any evidence linking cannabis use in a population and schizophrenia.

Another interesting finding of our analysis is what it would take to reduce the number of people being diagnosed with schizophrenia by targeting cannabis use. Our research estimates that, to prevent one episode of schizophrenia, [†]we would need to stop 5,000 men or 7,000 women aged 20 to 25 years from ever using the drug. This is obviously an impossible public-health challenge, and not a viable route towards reducing schizophrenia.

All of this was outlined in the ACMD's report. However, the government then summarily ignored it, which I believe has reinforced a popular impression that there is a far stronger causal relationship between cannabis and schizophrenia than there probably is. Many people with schizophrenia continue to take cannabis (even though they admit that it makes some symptoms worse), because it helps them to cope with major aspects of the disease like anxiety and tension, and lets them think more clearly; as with any medication, people decide whether the side effects are worth the benefit they gain. The situation we are seeing now is parents and doctors effectively blaming patients for their condition, sometimes even going so far as to claim they've brought the disease on themselves through their drug use. For most people this is highly unlikely to be true, and constitutes a hurtful new form of stigmatisation for a very distressed and damaged group.

Notes
Page

72 Henry VIII even passed a law requiring farmers to grow it!• *Marijuana - the first twelve thousand years*, Ernest Abel, Plenum Press, 1980. The decree stipulated that "for every 60 acres of arable land a farmer owned, a quarter acre was to be sown with hemp".

73 and the receptors it acts on are named *cannabis receptors*• *The Science of Marijuana*, Leslie I Iverson, Oxford University Press, 2000

74 "ma" in Chinese medicine• As above.

74 "bhang"• As above.

74 it was only popularised in Britain in the 1840s, by an army surgeon who had served in India• *Science and Technology - Ninth Report*, House of Lords Select Committee, URL-26, November 4th 1998

74 "when pure and administered carefully, it is one of the most valuable medicines we possess"• *On the therapeutic uses and toxic effects of cannabis indica*, JR Reynolds, The Lancet (1), March 1890

74 The condition that seems to benefit most commonly from the use of cannabis is multiple sclerosis (MS)• *Science and Technology - Ninth Report*, House of Lords Select Committee, URL-26, November 4th 1998

74 Cannabis also seems to have benefits in a number of other disorders, such as relieving the pain from a phantom limb among amputees, and preventing seizures in epileptics• As above.

75 many accounts of its helping inspire people's creativity• *The Effects of Cannabis Use on Creativity*, The Beckley Foundation Research Projects, URL-27, accessed December 12th 2011

75 scored 20 on our harm scale• *Drug harms in the UK: a multicriteria decision analysis*, David Nutt et al, ISCD, URL-16, November 1st 2010

75 Cannabis dependence occurs in about 10% of users• *Cannabis: classification and public health*, ACMD, April 2008

75 rimonabant, which block the effects of cannabis, can precipitate these withdrawal symptoms• *Antagonist-elicited cannabis withdrawal in humans*, DA Gorelick et al, Journal Clinical Psychopharmacology 31(5), 2011

76 In the UK in 2007/8, around 17,000 people were treated for cannabis addiction, half of them under 18• *Cannabis: classification and public health*, ACMD, April 2008

76 A study of US postal workers• As above.

76 Vietnamese gangs, who use illegal Vietnamese immigrants (some of them children) as workers in conditions of near-slave labour• As above.

78 Tests have shown that this doesn't actually increase THC levels in the brain• *The Science of Marijuana*, Leslie I. Iverson, Oxford University Press, 2000

78 THC levels were at one point as high as 21%, they soon dropped back down to 15%• *Cannabis: classification and public health*, ACMD, April 2008

79 overshadowed by the more potent painkilling properties of opium• *Indian Hemp and the Dope Fiends of Old England: A sociopolitical history of cannabis and the British Empire 1840–1928*, Sean Blanchard and Matthew J Atha, URL-28, 1994

80 Indian Hemp Drugs Commission report in 1894• *Indian Hemp Drugs Commission report in 1894*, Indian Hemp Drugs Commission, available online on the Medical History of British India website, URL-29, accessed December 7th 2011

80 In 1945 there were a total of 4 prosecutions for cannabis offences, and it wasn't until 1950 that the number of prosecutions for cannabis (86) outnumbered those for opium and other manufactured drugs (83).• *Indian Hemp and the Dope Fiends of Old England: A sociopolitical history of cannabis and the British Empire 1840–1928*, Sean Blanchard and Matthew J Atha, URL-28, 1994

81 The situation was very different in the USA• *Illegal drugs: a complete guide to their history, chemistry, use and abuse*, Paul M Ghalinger, Plume, 2003

82 diverting prescriptions from their doctors • *Necessity or nastiness? The hidden law denying cannabis for medicinal use*, David Nutt, URL-30, December 13th 2010

82 not to renew the medical licence on cannabis • *Science and Technology - Ninth Report*, House of Lords Select Committee, URL-26, November 4th 1998

83 the House of Lords Select Committee produced a report • As above.

84 the legal situation has become even more draconian in recent years • *Necessity or nastiness? The hidden law denying cannabis for medicinal use*, David Nutt, URL-30, December 13th 2010

84 James Brokenshire, who has insisted in Parliament • Cannabis Question in the House, URL-33, May 9th 2011, *"We do not recognise cannabis in its raw form to have any medicinal purposes; cannabis is a harmful drug. However, Sativex, a cannabis-based medicine, has been approved by the Medicines and Healthcare products Regulatory Agency as a safe and effective medicine for patients with multiple sclerosis."*

85 no varieties of hemp can be grown in the US • *Industrial Hemp in the US: Status and Market Potential*, United States Department of Agriculture Economic Research Service, URL-34, January 2000

85 requested the ACMD to review the status of cannabis for the third time • *Cannabis: classification and public health*, ACMD, April 2008

85 "Though statistics show that cannabis use has fallen significantly, there is real public concern about the potential mental-health effects of cannabis use, in particular the use of stronger forms of the drug, commonly known as skunk." • *Estimating Drug Harms: A Risky Business?*, David Nutt, URL-2, October 10th 2009

87 Figure 5.5 • after *Cannabis and schizophrenia: model projections of the impact of the rise in cannabis use on historical and future trends in schizophrenia in England and Wales*, URL-175, Matthew Hickman, Peter Vickerman, John Macleod, James Kirkbride and Peter B. Jones, Addiction, (102), 2007. Source: OCJS survey.

87 show that psychosis and schizophrenia are still on the decline • *Assessing the impact of cannabis use on trends in diagnosed schizophrenia in the United Kingdom from 1996 to 2005.*, M Frisher, I Crome, O Martino and P Croft, Schizophr Res 113: 123–128, 2009. And *Popular intoxicants: what lessons can be learned from the last 40 years of alcohol and cannabis regulation?*, Ruth Weissenborn and David J Nutt, Journal of Psychopharmacology, September 17th 2011

87 we would need to stop 5,000 men or 7,000 women • Michael Rawlins et al, *Cannabis: Classification and Public Health*, Home Office, URL-161, 2008

6 If alcohol were discovered today, would it be legal?

> *A TERRIFYING new "legal high" has hit our streets. Methyl-carbonol, known by the street name "wiz", is a clear liquid that causes cancers, liver problems, and brain disease, and is more toxic than ecstasy and cocaine. Addiction can occur after just one drink, and addicts will go to any lengths to get their next fix – even letting their kids go hungry or beating up their partners to obtain money. Casual users can go into blind RAGES when they're high, and police have reported a huge increase in crime where the drug is being used. Worst of all, drinks companies are adding "wiz" to fizzy drinks and advertising them to kids like they're plain Coca-Cola. Two or three teenagers die from it EVERY WEEK overdosing on a binge, and another TEN from having accidents caused by reckless driving. "Wiz" is a public menace – when will the Home Secretary think of the children and make this dangerous substance Class A?*

In the days following the publication of our harms paper, several newspapers ran headlines along the lines of "Professor Nutt says Alcohol Worse than Drugs", as though alcohol weren't a drug itself. This false distinction is a large part of the communication problem I encounter whenever I try to emphasise how harmful alcohol is. It has a separate language – you get "high" on drugs, but "drunk" on alcohol, drug addicts need a "fix" but alcoholics need a "drink". As I hope the satirical article above about alcohol shows (methylcarbonol is another chemical name for ethanol, which is the psychoactive part of alcohol), to think rationally about drugs policy we have to see alcohol in the same context as other drugs, not separately. Alcohol also has a lot to teach us about what *not* to do when a potentially lethal, habit-forming substance is legal.

We are currently facing a public-health crisis of immense proportions. The increase in harms caused by alcohol over the last 50 years in the UK is comparable to the Gin Craze in the early 18th century, when the urban poor of London were consuming a pint of gin a day per head on average. Recent annual statistics show:

- [†]Up to 40,000 alcohol-related deaths, including 350 just from acute alcohol poisoning and 8,000 from cirrhosis of the liver. More than a million hospital admissions in 2007/8 (including 13,000 under-18s), costing the NHS £2.7 billion.
- [†]7,000 road traffic accidents, including 500 deaths.
- [†]1.2 million violent incidents and 500,000 crimes, costing the police £7 billion.

In addition:

- [†]40% of domestic violence cases involve alcohol, as well as [†]50% of child protection cases.
- [†]3.5 million adults in the UK are addicted, and [†]up to 700,000 children live with a parent with a drink problem. [†]6,000 children a year are born with foetal alcohol syndrome each year.
- Globally, [†]the main burden of disease in 15–24 year-old males is due to alcohol, outweighing unsafe sex, illicit drug use, and physical accidents combined.
- The total economic cost has been calculated as [†]£30 billion a year – though some calculations estimate it may be as high as £55 billion.

Figure 6.1 [†]compares the death and disability burden in the EU, due to several causes, showing alcohol as the second most damaging.

The drinks industry responds to critiques like mine by saying that alcohol misuse affects only a "minority". Clearly, alcohol harms don't affect just a minority: they affect all of us – as victims of car crashes and street violence, as patients, as families of hazardous drinkers, and as taxpayers. Reducing these harms and associated costs is a huge public-health challenge that ought to be a top priority for our policy makers. Unfortunately, while the Labour government was talking "tough on drugs", trying to

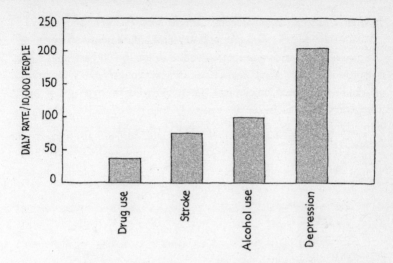

Figure 6.1: Costs of alcohol dependence, compared with other causes. ("DALY" is "disability-adjusted life year", a measure of overall disease burden, expressed as the number of years lost due to ill-health, disability or early death.)

score political points by making cannabis Class B, banning mephedrone and exaggerating the harms of ecstasy, they missed the growing epidemic around the most harmful drug of all – or more accurately just looked the other way.

How the drinks industry influences alcohol policy

The drinks industry is one of the most powerful industrial groups in the UK today, and spends huge sums of money on maintaining its privileged relationship with our lawmakers. Political lobbying takes place largely in secret. Even so, the †Labour government's 2004 Alcohol Harm Reduction Strategy shows clear evidence of the influence of the drinks industry, because it focused on the measures the industry had recommended (such as information campaigns and education) and ignored the measures recommended by the Chief Medical Officer (such as minimum pricing). In fact, the House of Commons Health Committee itself commented on this in its 2009–2010 report on alcohol: [†]*"we are concerned that Government policies are much closer to, and too influenced by those of the drinks industry and the supermarkets than those of expert health professionals such as the Royal College of Physicians or the CMO [Chief Medical Officer]"*.

Like the tobacco lobby before it, the industry has taken proactive steps to protect the public image of its product even as the evidence about the harm done by alcohol has become incontrovertible. The European Centre for Monitoring Alcohol Marketing recently published a report called *The Seven Key Messages of the Alcohol Industry*, which summarises the sorts of messages the industry uses to try and influence alcohol policy:

1. Consuming alcohol is normal, common, healthy and very responsible.
2. The damage done by alcohol is caused by a small group of deviants who cannot handle alcohol.
3. Normal adult non-drinkers do not, in fact, exist.
4. Ignore the fact that alcohol is a harmful and addictive chemical substance (ethanol) for the body.
5. Alcohol problems can only be solved when all parties work together.
6. Alcohol marketing is not harmful. It is simply intended to assist the consumer in selecting a certain product or brand.
7. Education about responsible use is the best method to protect society from alcohol problems.

These messages are at best distortions of reality, and at worst outright lies. Their intention is to misdirect policymakers away from measures that will actually reduce harm, and towards policies that will allow the industry to continue to make huge profits at the expense of public health and well-being. Let's look at each of their claims in turn.

1a. Consuming alcohol is normal

It's certainly true that most societies throughout history have brewed some sort of alcoholic drink, and that this has been part of the human diet for so long that many of us are genetically adapted to consume alcohol.

When ethanol breaks down in the body it produces acetaldehyde, a substance even more toxic than alcohol, which needs to be oxidised to avoid unpleasant and dangerous effects. People from ethnic groups who don't have a history of alcohol use – such as Native Americans, Inuit, and many Chinese – often have a form of the ALDH2 enzyme (the enzyme that breaks down acetaldehyde) which is less effective at this oxidation process, leading to high levels of acetaldehyde in their system when they drink. The resulting facial flushing, nausea, headaches and general discomfort largely outweigh the pleasant effects of intoxication, and by and large these groups drink less alcohol than groups who have a more active form of the enzyme (as most Europeans, Africans and South Americans do), and suffer less alcohol addiction and liver disease.

So, drinking alcohol is "normal", in a sense – people who possess the high-activity variant of the ALDH2 enzyme, come from a long line of people whose bodies adapted to consuming and breaking down alcohol. Indeed, until the 1850s weak beer was often "healthy": it was the safest thing to drink, because most water was contaminated with viruses or bacteria. However, in the past most of what was drunk was mostly relatively low strength beer and wine, and its consumption was surrounded by custom and ritual to mitigate its social harms.

The other, more recent, history of alcohol is one of disruption and damage, where societies that are unfamiliar with its effects suffer hugely when new types of alcohol appear, particularly if they are aggressively marketed. From the Gin Craze in Britain in the 18th century, to the enormous rates of alcoholism on Native American reserves in the USA, there are dozens of examples of societies unable to cope socially and medically with the drug. We're at a similar point now in the UK: the access people have to cheap, high-strength alcohol is almost unprecedented, and binge drinking of the sort we see today is something our ancestors would rarely have been able to indulge in even if they'd wanted to. Teenagers being encouraged to drink themselves to death every day is not what any society should consider "normal".

1b. Consuming alcohol is healthy

What about the health benefits of alcohol? The drug does have some positive psychological effects, and it can be calming for some people with anxiety disorders (see Case Study 1 below) although with heavy use the effects of withdrawal will start to make them even more anxious when they're sober.

Case Study 1

I was called out on a home visit to see a man in his late 40s with severe agoraphobia (the fear of going out). He had been drinking heavily all his life, and was now dying from cirrhosis and the damage alcohol had done to his nerves. He had been diagnosed as an alcoholic, but the reason he drank was to control his extreme anxiety: he told me he had to drink four cans of lager to be able to get to his Alcoholics Anonymous meetings, and one can just to be able to brave going outside to cut the grass. His anxiety disorder pre-dated the drinking, and, having been given no other help, he felt forced to self-medicate with alcohol. But as soon as he started drinking regularly, all the health practitioners he saw identified his primary problem as alcoholism, and no one would treat the underlying anxiety while he kept drinking. I treated him with SSRI antidepressants which help with anxiety disorders.

Physiologically, alcohol's benefits have never been proven, but the idea that low levels of drinking are protective is a pervasive myth – and a very useful one for the industry. We know that, [†]for a particular group of people (middle-aged men), those that drink small amounts, particularly of red wine, have slightly lower levels of heart disease than those who don't drink at all. However, this may be because this group have more-healthy lifestyles, or because of the "sick teetotaller effect" – where many people give up alcohol because they are ill (perhaps from some other disease); their worse health outcomes may have nothing to do with whether or not they drink, but do make the health statistics of non-drinkers appear worse. To know for sure if alcohol is actually preventing heart disease, we would need to do a randomised trial where some of this group drink no alcohol, others drink it in small amounts and others drink more heavily. Until this experiment has been done we don't have *proof* that alcohol has health benefits.

As I've written before, there is [†]no such thing as a safe level of alcohol consumption. Alcohol is a toxin that kill cells and organisms, which is why we use it to preserve food and sterilise needles. Acetaldehyde, produced when the body breaks down alcohol, is even more toxic, and any food or drink contaminated with the amount of acetaldehyde that a unit of alcohol produces would immediately be banned as having an unacceptable health risk.

Although rare, alcohol addiction after a single drink does happen in a small proportion of cases, as you can read in Case Study 2; since we can't predict who those people will be, any exposure to alcohol runs the risk of producing addiction in some users. And apart from the possible cardiovascular benefits of low intake for some middle-aged men, for [†]all other diseases associated with alcohol the risks rise inexorably with intake. This isn't to say that I think nobody should ever drink at all – I drink myself, and enjoy it. But I understand that there are always risks involved, and I certainly don't drink for the good of my health.

Case Study 2

I was taken to see a man in his late 30s who had been admitted to hospital to dry out. He'd been through problematic withdrawal several times, and had had seizures in the past when trying to dry out. I asked him when his drinking began. He said he was given his first can of beer at age seven when he was out fishing with his dad, and he immediately felt that the person he became when under the influence of alcohol was his real self; "for the first time in my life, I felt normal". He probably belongs to a minority of people who are biologically programmed to have very strong liking for alcohol, and are highly likely to become alcoholics. Hopefully in the future we will be able to identify these people before they start drinking, so they know to avoid the drug, and we may develop medications to help them feel normal without alcohol.

1c. Consuming alcohol is responsible

"Responsible drinking" is another industry favourite. It's a very curious phrase, considering the drug's actual effects. Alcohol is a depressant (similar to GHB, and benzodiazepines like Valium) which, if taken at high enough doses, will produce amnesia, sedation and eventually death. It stimulates the GABA receptors in the brain, reducing anxiety and motor coordination, and blocks [†]specific glutamate receptors, switching off the parts of your brain that keep you alert and awake, and switching on the parts that make you drowsy and tired.

Alcohol also indirectly stimulates the noradrenaline circuit, producing some stimulating effects. This is what creates the noisy energy we associate with drunkenness, even though the drug is a depressant. Some interesting recent research showed that [†]alcohol interferes with our ability to recognise emotions in facial expressions, which may be part of the reason drunk people are so quick to take offence and start fights. The overall effects of increasing GABA and noradrenaline in the brain are disinhibition, decreased concern for social codes and standards of behaviour, an increase in risk taking and disregard for long-term consequences. I'm sure the majority of the 40 million drinkers in this country are people who take their responsibilities seriously in everyday life, but almost all of them – with the possible exception of addicts in withdrawal – will be more responsible when they're sober!

2. The damage done by alcohol is caused by a small group of deviants who cannot handle alcohol

The statistics on page 92 show that millions of people, *not* a tiny minority, suffer harm from their own alcohol consumption, or cause harm to others. Alcohol dependence is on the rise, with the attendant social damage and ruined lives, and binge drinking is killing hundreds of people a year as well as causing cirrhosis in patients as young as their early 20s. But it's very important to understand that much of the surge in harms is actually among people who don't engage in these extreme behaviours. It is the everyday drinking of people who have come to see alcohol as an essential part of life rather than the luxury it used to be, that has created a spike in cancers and stomach problems, and will see †liver disease match heart disease as the leading cause of death in the UK by 2020. This new habitual daily consumption has been made possible because alcohol is now only a third the cost relative to income than it was in the 1950s, and particularly because of the availability of cheap liquor in supermarkets.

3. Normal adult non-drinkers do not, in fact, exist

The drinks industry wants to portray itself as serving an important social function, and remind governments of how unpopular any measures to restrict access to alcohol will be. The existence of non-drinkers obviously threatens this portrayal of society, so the industry tends to dismiss them as having something wrong with them. While some teetotallers *are* recovering alcoholics, many others have made a positive choice not to drink. Some don't drink because there is alcoholism in the family and they know they are at increased risk of becoming dependent if they start. Others, particularly sports-people, know that alcohol impairs performance, so they never touch it – David Beckham is teetotal, for example. And, of course, many people avoid the drug for religious or cultural reasons. These are all perfectly valid choices, yet non-drinkers are often heavily pressured to consume alcohol in order to fit in with others. This message is constantly reinforced in the press, on TV, and in alcohol advertising.

4a. Ignore the fact that alcohol is a harmful substance for the body

Far from being safe, there is no other drug which is so damaging to so many different organ systems in the body. Figure 6.2 illustrates how alcohol can harm almost every part of the body through its toxicity alone. (The Figure doesn't show the other physical damage caused by falls, road traffic accidents and violence). Most other drugs cause damage primarily in one or two areas – heart problems from cocaine, or urinary tract problems from ketamine. Alcohol is harmful almost everywhere.

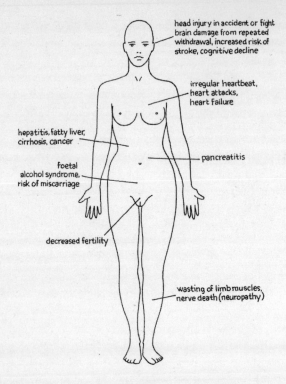

Figure 6.2: Alcohol damages almost every organ system in the body.

4b. Ignore the fact that alcohol is addictive

Alcohol is not the most addictive drug, but its widespread availability and social acceptability make becoming dependent more likely. This social context also makes relapse after treatment highly likely, as Case Study 3 shows. It can be hard for anyone, let alone an addict, to refuse a drink when it's offered socially. [†]About a quarter of the adult population of the UK drink more than the recommended weekly limit; 6% of men and 2% of women are "harmful drinkers", where damage to health is likely, and levels are higher still in Scotland. As with many other drugs, dependent users suffer withdrawal symptoms when they stop. The withdrawal syndrome for alcohol is characterised by tremors,

Drugs – without the hot air, David Nutt

nausea, extreme irritability, and sometimes fits and delirium, which can be life-threatening.

Case Study 3

A 28-year-old man had been in for treatment which had gone well – he had dried out and seemed in good shape when he left us. A few months later he was readmitted. I asked him why he had relapsed and he said that he'd been walking past an off-licence and had had such an uncontrollable urge to drink he'd walked in and drunk a whole bottle of vodka right there in the shop. Helping people stop drinking is relatively easy; avoiding relapse, especially when cheap high-strength alcohol is available on every street corner, is much more difficult.

5. Alcohol problems can only be solved when all parties work together

The drinks industry wants to portray itself as having the same aims and interests as people who want alcohol policy to be guided by a concern for public health. But there is a fundamental conflict of interest: however much the industry wants to pretend otherwise, you can't reduce harm without reducing the amount people drink, whereas companies looking to maximise profits need to sell as much alcohol as possible. There is a lot of evidence that the drinks industry relies upon hazardous drinking as a major source of income. In fact, it has been calculated that if everyone who drinks more than the recommended daily limit started drinking moderately there would be a †drop in total alcohol consumption of 40% – equivalent to over £13 billion in sales. However much the industry talks about taking the harms seriously, nothing can change the fact that their success is indirectly related to the amount of damage they inflict on society at large.

This is not to say that they bring no benefit to society at all – brewers contribute billions every year in tax revenue, and the industry does provide a lot of jobs. Pubs in particular are important social spaces and local employers, but they've seen their profits plummet in recent years as a result of the cut-price alcohol available from supermarkets and off-licences. "Working together" implies that everyone can win, when in fact politicians need to weigh up the different interests involved, and bring in policies that will produce the best outcomes for society as a whole, even if that means that some parties have to lose out.

In practice, what the industry means by "working together" is bringing in voluntary codes rather than statutory regulation – solving problems through rules that the industry *chooses* to comply with, rather than laws which they *must* comply with. These are supposed to be easier to implement and more flexible than going down the legal route. However, evidence from across the world shows that the [†]voluntary codes adopted by drinks industries are essentially ineffective at reducing alcohol harms – they tend to focus on the wrong sort of interventions, and are routinely ignored by signatory companies anyway. This was recognised with smoking and the tobacco industry, and is equally true of those who profit from alcohol.

6. Alcohol marketing is not harmful. It is simply intended to assist the consumer in selecting a certain product or brand

The drinks industry spends around [†]£800 million a year on advertising, marketing, sponsorship, contests and special promotions. While the most important factors determining consumption are price and availability, marketing does have a demonstrable impact on *levels* of drinking, not just the brands people choose to drink.

This is particularly true with young people and a number of studies have concluded that marketing communications do have a marked effect on consumption. A recent British Medical Association (BMA) publication, [†]*Under the Influence*, revealed many of the techniques the drinks industry employs to target a younger audience, including email campaigns with embedded film clips advertising alcohol, Facebook links and texts going direct to people's phones.

The industry claim that their advertising is aimed at providing information and choice, but there is a powerful symbolism to the sheer volume of advertising that people are exposed to on a daily basis. To quote the BMA: *"the fact that promotion is allowed, ubiquitous and heavily linked to mainstream cultural phenomena, communicates a legitimacy and status to alcohol that belies the harms associated with its use. It also severely limits the effectiveness of any public health message."* There's a lot of evidence that the more common and acceptable consuming alcohol is seen to be, the more people will drink, and this cultural context is especially influential on young people. All this further entrenches the false division between alcohol and illegal drugs, persuades people that consuming alcohol is safe, and makes realistic discussions of the harm alcohol causes very difficult.

7. Education about responsible use is the best method to protect society from alcohol problems

It is useful for the drinks industry to emphasise the value of education, because it takes the focus off regulation: if how much a person drinks is just their individual choice, then there's no need to control how much alcohol they have access to. As well as being implausible with a drug like alcohol that dissolves one's self-control, there is also extensive evidence gathered by the WHO from around the world, showing that [†]merely providing information and education without bringing in other policy measures doesn't change people's drinking behaviour. At best, they are a waste of money – though in the UK the sums involved (a few million pounds a year) are pitifully small anyway. At worst, especially when these education programmes are funded by the industry, they can reinforce heavy drinking by improving people's opinions of the industry. This is especially worrying in the UK, as from [†]1989 to 2006 the drinks-industry-run Portman Group was funding and delivering many of the alcohol-awareness campaigns in this country.

Of course I believe that informing people about the harms done by drugs has an important role to play in reducing those harms – that's why I've written this book – but it's not enough on its own. When it comes to an addictive substance that impairs our judgement, we can't rely on people cutting down the amount they use, just because they have a rational understanding of its harms. If the product is freely available, being aggressively marketed all around them, and changes their brain to make self-control nearly impossible, they need other sorts of interventions too.

How can we reduce the harm done by alcohol?

So what *can* we do? As the title of this chapter suggests, one approach would be to ban alcohol altogether. While this would be consistent with policies towards other drugs, we know from historical examples that it would be laden with perverse consequences. Where prohibition has been tried in the West, most famously †in the USA from 1920 to 1933, medical harms such as deaths from liver cirrhosis were reduced over the population as a whole, but the policies were considered failures. This was because the social harms of the resulting "bootleg" alcohol market put so much money and power into the hands of criminal gangs that law and order broke down. The effects were so severe they led to the repeal of prohibition. Even in the Islamic world, where the religion's long-standing ban on the drug makes prohibition politically possible, the use and abuse of alcohol is well known.

Banning alcohol outright would be an extreme and probably counter-productive measure, but fortunately there are other options available to governments. I'd like to counter the drinks industry's seven key messages with seven suggestions of my own for reducing alcohol harms:

A. Increase the price.
B. Restrict availability.
C. Make alcohol a national health priority.
D. Make alcohol dependence a priority for the
   National Treatment Agency.
E. Stop people binge drinking.
F. Save lives on the road.
G. Provide alternatives.

A. Increase the price

In the 1950s, alcohol was three times the price relative to income as it is now, and we drank half as much. Evidence from across the world shows that the †price of alcohol determines use for almost everyone, with the possible exception of severely-dependent drinkers. The government should triple the cost of alcohol progressively over five years, through a minimum price per unit, or through increased taxation. I prefer the second option because it delivers more money back to the public purse, helping to offset the costs of the harm caused by the drug. If we did go down the minimum pricing route, a simple way to calculate it would be to charge the same amount in a shop as the average price in a pub.

We already tax different classes of alcohol differently, but with the invention of super-strength lagers and ciders we need to extend this principle and start taxing drinks according to their alcohol content. It makes no sense for an 8% alcohol-content cider to be taxed at a quarter of the rate of a 12% wine; a can of 8% lager should cost twice as much as a 4% can, and four times as much as a 2% can. Discounted alcohol in Happy Hours and "all you can drink for £20" offers should be banned, and subsidies removed for bars in government-supported organisations, such as universities.

Some people might argue that increasing the price of alcohol will unfairly affect the poor – but many of the poor are poor because they're addicted to alcohol and tobacco. Increasing the price of cigarettes has significantly reduced demand, and there is every reason to think this would be the case for alcohol as well. Since alcohol-related damage already costs each taxpayer £1,000 a year, tripling the price and reducing the harm by two thirds would save everyone £666, making up for the price increase over the bar. Anyone that would be financially worse off under this plan is drinking at a dangerous level anyway. It's possible that this could lead to higher levels of smuggling, although with tobacco there is †no clear relationship between levels of taxation and levels of smuggling (in fact, countries with the lowest levels of taxation have historically had the most smuggling). Effective border controls have substantially reduced the amount of contraband tobacco coming into the UK, even as the price has been rising, and there's no reason to think that this couldn't work just as effectively for alcohol.

B. Restrict availability

The availability of a drug has a strong relationship with the number of people who will become addicted to it. We need to reverse the trend of people drinking large amounts in the home or at all hours in licensed venues. Repealing the 24-hour Licensing Act so that pubs and bars close at 11pm would be part of this, alongside adopting the Swedish model where any drinks over 3% have to be sold from licensed shops with limited opening hours. With supermarkets no longer able to sell high strength, cut-price alcohol at any hour of the day, people are more likely to do their drinking in pubs, rather than at home or on the street. Pubs are good places to consume alcohol because they are sociable spaces where intoxication can be monitored, and young people can learn to drink more responsibly. (However, it's worth pointing out that in recent years we have seen unsavoury developments in bar practices which encourage dangerous drinking. These include reducing seating so people have to stand, special cut price and "all-you-can-drink" offers, and happy hours with 2-for-the-price-of-1 deals. These encourage irresponsible and heavy drinking and should be banned.)

C. Make alcohol a national health priority

We know that public-health campaigns really do work: when the current Health Secretary Andrew Lansley cut the funding on anti-smoking campaigns in 2010, †the number of people contacting the NHS to help them quit fell noticeably. Public campaigns, to make people aware of the damage alcohol does, and make excessive drinking unfashionable, would help people reduce their intake. All alcohol advertising should be banned, and drinks containing alcohol should have warning notices similar to those on cigarette packets, containing information about its physical risks and social and economic costs.

Education about the dangers of alcohol should start in primary school. However, we already know from research that, †on its own, lecturing

Drugs – without the hot air, David Nutt

teenagers about drug harms is not very effective, and may do more harm than good. A more creative approach is a [†]model that has been tested successfully in East Sussex. This focuses on the drinks industry itself. Students are given information about the way the industry ignores its own voluntary codes, the influence it has on the public-health message around alcohol, and the political agendas surrounding alcohol consumption, along with the costs of drinking to users and society. The students are then asked to make up their own minds about the issues. We should encourage wider use of this sort of education.

D. Make alcohol dependence a priority for the National Treatment Agency

There are a number of promising lines of research into pharmacological substitutes and therapies, which can work well alongside psychological treatments like cognitive behavioural therapy (CBT) and Alcoholics Anonymous. The pleasant effects of alcohol are caused by the release of natural opioids; substances such as acamprosate and naltrexone block these, making the experience less pleasurable, and so might help in treatment. Some recent research has found that building up tolerance to alcohol also results in a [†]huge increase in tolerance to GHB: where an alcoholic might be able to take three times as much as a non-alcoholic without overdosing, they can tolerate much more GHB. Although the mechanism is unclear, it may be that GHB could act as a safer alternative for those severely dependent on alcohol, as they'd be less likely to kill themselves. (But it is important to note that for people who are *not* tolerant to alcohol, GHB/GBL taken with alcohol is very dangerous – because the two drugs reinforce each other's respiratory-depressant effects.)

GHB is used in Italy and Austria to treat alcoholism. The potential as an alcohol treatment of another drug, baclofen, that acts on GABA receptors, has been discussed by a recovering alcoholic, Olivier Ameisen, in his book *The End of My Addiction*, and [†]a number of doctors are now using this drug to treat alcoholics, particularly those with liver disease. There should be more funding for research in this area.

E. Stop people binge drinking

To stop binge drinking we need a cultural change. It's very difficult to achieve this through regulation, but we could start by banning companies who run events at which reckless levels of drinking routinely occur, such as the student event promoter, Carnage UK. The dangers of these events are well-recognised by public services; as the National Union of Students' vice-president for Welfare said, [†]"Any organised bar crawl that has an ambulance following behind it clearly has something deeply wrong." While it would be hard to regulate private groups, drinking games and pub crawls should be banned in government-supported organisations like university sports and social clubs, and financial support removed if they continue to host them.

There are other simple steps we can take. Wine should be sold in 125ml glasses again, rather than the 175ml or even 250ml ones which have crept in. This is especially important for women, who often drink wine; women's higher proportion of body fat means they experience about twice the effect per unit of alcohol compared with men. The measures suggested above to reduce cheap alcohol sales from supermarkets are likely to reduce "pre-loading" (drinking large amounts before going out to pubs or bars). We should enforce the law that makes serving drunk customers illegal, and have breathalysers available to back up the judgement of bar staff. If someone's blood alcohol concentration is over 150 mg/100ml they shouldn't be served until they've sobered up a bit.

F. Save lives on the road

Decrease the drink-driving limit to 40 mg/100 ml in blood, assess people properly when they're caught, and revoke their licence if they flout DVLA guidance to be assessed as fit to drive again. Encourage the wider use in cars of alcohol detectors that won't allow the car to start if the driver is over the limit. [†]A large number of road deaths are among young people, and raising the drinking age to 21 would almost certainly reduce them. Road deaths [†]declined by 11% after the USA did this in the 1990s.

G. Provide alternatives

Make it law that all alcohol outlets have to sell non-alcoholic beers and lagers as well, so that people who like the taste of these drinks can experience it without the risk of intoxication. The quality of these is improving, and although some seasoned drinkers say they prefer the taste of alcoholic versions, this is mostly the result of repeated conditioning to the alcohol which is exactly the effect we need to reverse. Non-alcoholic drinks should be cheaper than their alcoholic equivalent, and made obviously available in shops and in all bars.

Another route to explore (which has formed part of my academic research), is investigating less dangerous alternatives to alcohol, to provide some of the pleasurable effects of mild to moderate inebriation without the harms. The active ingredient would probably be a benzodiazepine (there are thousands) which could be produced as a liquid and added to other sorts of flavoured drinks. Ideally, it would be impossible to get drunk on, just producing a moderate buzz with no increase in effects at higher doses. It would also come with an antidote – a "sober pill" that could be popped at the end of the night to reverse the effect of the drug, so that people could get home safely, even if they were driving.

Conclusion

Realistically this kind of policy-making is probably a long way off. Many of the measures I've suggested would be profoundly unpopular, and would require real leadership from government – and a willingness to stand up to criticism from both the drinks industry and the tabloids. The House of Commons Health Committee summarised the failures of many different areas of government to take action on alcohol harms in stark terms in its [†]2009–10 report:

> "DCMS [Department of Culture, Media and Sport] has been particularly close to the drinks industry. The interests of large pub chains and the promotion of the "night-time" economy have taken priority; Ofcom, the ASA [Advertising Standards Authority] and the Portman Group preside over an advertising and marketing

regime which is failing to adequately protect young people. OFT [The Office of Fair Trading] shows a blinkered obsession with competition heedless of concerns for public health. The Treasury for many years has pursued a policy of making spirits cheaper in real terms. Collectively, government has failed to address the alcohol problem."

The report gives little grounds for optimism, and yet the harms of alcohol are becoming so severe that it's inevitable that a government in the not-too-distant future will have to start considering serious harm-reduction measures of the kind I have suggested. And we do have a precedent for this kind of action in the public-health response to tobacco. Almost all the measures brought in, from banning smoking in the workplace to health warnings on packets, faced substantial opposition at first, but in time came to be seen as necessary and desirable by the majority of people.

To get the buy-in of the public, politicians can lead the way by reducing their own use of alcohol. They can also declare any association with the drinks industry, in recognition of the fact that regularly using the drug or consorting with its promoters may distort their objectivity in making laws about it. They can close the government's wine cellar and stop subsidising alcohol in the Houses of Parliament, so they pay the same prices as everyone else when they drink. Once people see MPs taking the harms of alcohol seriously, they may be less hostile to the measures I've suggested. If any government is serious about being "tough on drugs", they need to be tough on the most harmful drug of all: alcohol.

Notes
Page

92 Up to 40,000 alcohol-related deaths, including 350 just from acute alcohol poisoning and 8,000 from cirrhosis of the liver. More than a million hospital admissions in 2007/8 (including 13,000 under-18s), costing the NHS £2.7 billion• *Alcohol: First Report of Session 2009–10*, House of Commons Health Committee, December 10th 2009

92 7,000 road traffic accidents, including 500 deaths• *Chief Medical Officer 150th annual report*, Liam Donaldson, 2008

Drugs – without the hot air, David Nutt

92 1.2 million violent incidents and 500,000 crimes, costing the police £7 billion• *Alcohol: First Report of Session 2009–10*, House of Commons Health Committee, December 10th 2009

92 40% of domestic violence cases involve alcohol• As above.

92 50% of child protection cases• *Swept under the carpet: children affected by parental alcohol misuse*, Alcohol Concern, URL-35, October 2010

92 3.5 million adults in the UK are addicted• *Alcohol: First Report of Session 2009–10*, House of Commons Health Committee, December 10th 2009

92 up to 700,000 children live with a parent with a drink problem• *Swept under the carpet: children affected by parental alcohol misuse*, Alcohol Concern, URL-35, October 2010

92 6,000 children a year are born with foetal alcohol syndrome• *Alcohol: First Report of Session 2009–10*, URL-162, House of Commons Health Committee, December 10th 2009

92 the main burden of disease in 15–24 year-old males• *Global burden of disease in young people aged 10–24 years: a systematic analysis*, URL-163, Fiona M Gore, et al, Lancet, June 2011

92 £30 billion a year – though some calculations estimate it may be as high as £55 billion• As above.

92 compares the death and disability burden in the EU,• *The size and burden of mental disorders and other disorders of the brain in Europe 2010*, URL-164, ECNP/EBC Report 2011

93 Labour government's 2004 Alcohol Harm Reduction Strategy shows clear evidence of the influence of the drinks industry• As above.

94 "we are concerned that Government policies are much closer to, and too influenced by those of the drinks industry and the supermarkets• *Alcohol: First Report of Session 2009–10*, URL-162, House of Commons Health Committee, December 10th 2009

96 for a particular group of people (middle-aged men), those that drink small amounts, particularly of red wine, have slightly lower levels of heart disease• *Alcohol: no ordinary commodity*, Thomas Babor et al, Oxford University Press, 2003

97 no such thing as a safe level of alcohol consumption• *There is no such thing as a safe level of alcohol consumption*, David Nutt, URL-36, March 7th 2011

97 all other diseases associated with alcohol the risks rise inexorably with intake• *Alcohol: no ordinary commodity*, Thomas Babor et al, Oxford University Press, 2003

98 specific glutamate receptors• These are the NMDA glutamate receptors.

98 alcohol interferes with our ability to recognise emotions in facial expressions• *Effects of acute alcohol consumption on processing of perceptual cues of emotional expression*, AS Attwood, C Ohlson, CP Benton, IS Penton-Voak, MR Munafò, Journal of Psychopharmacology 23(1), 2009

99 liver disease match heart disease as the leading cause of death in the UK by 2020• *I am not a Prohibitionist*, David Nutt, URL-37, November 5th 2010

100 About a quarter of the adult population of the UK drink more than the recommended weekly limit• *Statistics on Alcohol: England 2010*, NHS Information Centre, URL-38, 2010

101 drop in total alcohol consumption of 40%• *Alcohol: First Report of Session 2009–10*, House of Commons Health Committee, December 10th 2009

102 voluntary codes adopted by drinks industries are essentially ineffective at reducing alcohol harms• As above.

102 £800 million a year on advertising, marketing, sponsorship, contests and special promotions• *The seven key messages of the alcohol industry*, European Centre for Monitoring Alcohol Marketing, URL-39, February 2011

102 *Under the Influence*• British Medical Association, URL-40, September 7th 2009

103 merely providing information and education without bringing in other policy measures doesn't change people's drinking behaviour• *Alcohol: First Report of Session 2009–10*, House of Commons Health Committee, December 10th 2009

103 1989 to 2006 the drinks-industry-run Portman Group was funding and delivering many of the alcohol-awareness campaigns in this country• As above.

104 in the USA from 1920 to 1933, medical harms such as deaths from liver cirrhosis were reduced over the population as a whole, but the policies were considered failures• *Lessons from Alcohol Policy for Drug Policy*, Harry G. Levine and Craig Reinarman, URL-41, 2004

105 price of alcohol determines use for almost everyone• *Alcohol: First Report of Session 2009–10*, House of Commons Health Committee, December 10th 2009

105 no clear relationship between levels of taxation and levels of smuggling• *Cough Up*, Policy Exchange, URL-42, March 18th 2010

106 the number of people contacting the NHS to help them quit fell• *Andrew Lansley forced to make U-turn on public health campaign cuts*, Daniel Boffey, URL-43, May 28th 2011

Drugs – without the hot air, David Nutt

106 on its own, lecturing teenagers about drug harms is not very effective, and may do more harm than good• *Alcohol: First Report of Session 2009–10*, House of Commons Health Committee, December 10th 2009

107 model that has been tested successfully in East Sussex• *Teaching the tricks of the liquor trade*, Paul Myles, URL-44, January 19th 2011

107 huge increase in tolerance to GHB• *Cross-tolerance to ethanol and γ-hydroxy-butyric acid*, Giancarlo Colombo et al, Alcoholism: Clinical and Experimental Research, Volume 23 (10), October 1999

107 a number of doctors are now using this drug to treat alcoholics,• *Substitution therapy for alcoholism: time for a reappraisal?*, URL-165, J Chick and DJ Nutt, Journal of Psychopharmacology, July 8th, 2011

108 "Any organised bar crawl that has an ambulance following behind it clearly has something deeply wrong."• *Student pub crawls face ban amid backlash over drunken disorder*, Amelia Hill, URL-45, November 8th 2009.

108 A large number of road deaths are among young people• *Drinking and Driving*, Institute of Alcohol Studies Fact Sheet, URL-46, October 19th 2010

108 declined by 11% after the USA did this in the 1990s• *Minimum drinking age of 21 cuts road deaths*, Reuters, URL-47, July 1st 2008

109 2009–10 report• *Alcohol: First Report of Session 2009–10*, House of Commons Health Committee, December 10th 2009

7 "Meow meow" – should mephedrone have been banned?

"Meow meow"

In March 2010, I was lecturing in Barcelona when I got a call from CNN, and an American down the other end asked: "Where's Scunthorpe?" This was the first I heard about the deaths of Louis Wainwright and Nicholas Smith, two teenagers who had died after a night of heavy drinking and taking illegal drugs. Humberside police had immediately called an international press conference in which they linked the deaths with mephedrone, a legal "designer drug" which is chemically similar to amphetamine, and which the tabloids had nicknamed "meow meow". CNN wanted a quote from me, but as I knew nothing about the case all I could say was that it would be very surprising for mephedrone to have been the cause of the boys' deaths, and we needed to be sure of the evidence before we jumped to conclusions.

From the beginning, it seemed unlikely that mephedrone was responsible. The boys had been drinking heavily, and had died when they stopped breathing; if anything, taking a stimulant would have been protective. But as it turned out, [†]they hadn't taken mephedrone at all. As the toxicology report eventually showed, they had actually mixed alcohol and the heroin substitute methadone – possibly by mistake, because of their similar sounding names. As the boys tragically discovered, mixing depressants like alcohol with opiates is extremely dangerous. (This also turned out to have been the cause of death for 18-year-old [†]Joslyne Cockburn, who died the weekend after.) The fact that the new legal high had nothing to do with either case didn't stop the police, the media, or politicians from using them as evidence for why it needed to be banned.

The media storm around mephedrone had begun with the death of Gabrielle Price, a 14-year-old from Brighton who collapsed after allegedly taking it at a party, although she was eventually found to have [†]died from bronchopneumonia caused by a streptococcal A infection and hadn't taken any drugs at all. Extreme stories of mephedrone's harmful effects began to fill the papers. The *Sun* reproduced an account from a message board in which someone claimed to have [†]ripped off his own scrotum while high on mephedrone, [†]though this turned out to have been made up. More and more deaths were linked to it, long before confirmation from coroners that it was responsible, or had even been taken by the person who died. Quite aside from the ethical issues of whipping up hysteria with fictional articles, an analysis of internet activity clearly shows that every time a big story was published, interest in the drug increased – more people searched for information, and sales went up. Far from protecting people by exposing the truth, [†]the media through publicising the drug were contributing to its astronomical rise in use (Figure 7.1).

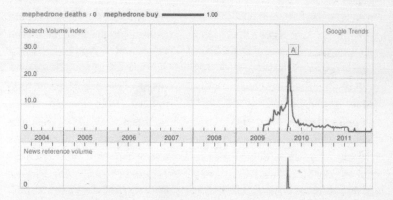

Figure 7.1: Google Trends for March 2010, showing how peak of search volume for "mephedrone" (top) coincided with media coverage of mephedrone deaths (bottom).

What is mephedrone and why is it called plant food?

Mephedrone is the common name for 4-methylmethcathinone. This is a synthetic derivative of cathinone, which is the active ingredient in the East African plant khat. (See box *The original cathinone: khat* on page 126.) Mephedrone was first synthesised in 1929, and largely forgotten until the early 2000s, when some [†]Israeli scientists working for an insecticide company started experimenting with cathinones. They were looking for a more ecological way to protect plants and searching for a chemical that would disrupt the brain activity of greenfly and make them easier for ladybirds to catch. Mephedrone did this to some extent, and so was used for a few years as a horticultural product. However, third-party companies soon discovered its psychoactive effects and started buying up hundreds of kilos to sell as a party drug in Israel, where it became widely used. Because of mephedrone's origin as a plant protector, it got the nickname "plant food", although calling it that and labelling it "not for human consumption" also proved useful for avoiding food safety standards. As well as its media nickname "meow-meow", mephedrone has many other street-names, including Drone, M-cat, and bubbles.

Mephedrone is usually sold as a white or off-white powder, although sometimes it comes as a pill. It's water-soluble, so it can be injected. However, it is too unstable to be smoked. It is usually snorted (for more short-lived effects), or swallowed (when the effect lasts longer but has less of a rush). Although we don't know many of the specifics about its action on the brain, it is chemically similar to amphetamine, and it's likely that it works like other stimulants, promoting the release of dopamine, noradrenaline, and possibly serotonin.

The drug was widely used in Israel until it was banned in 2007. It was banned partly because the authorities were concerned about conscripts taking it while they were doing their time in the army, though in the years that it was legal and popular no deaths were reported. It caught people's attention in the UK in 2009, and there was an extremely rapid increase in the number of users over the second half of the year. A [†]survey of Tayside schoolchildren and university students in February 2010 showed

Drugs – without the hot air, David Nutt

that 20% of them had tried it, and in late 2009 a survey of readers of *Mixmag* magazine found it was the [†]fourth most popular drug amongst clubbers (cannabis, ecstasy and cocaine being the most popular). Its subjective effects seem to be partway between ecstasy and cocaine – users say it increases their self-confidence and makes them more talkative (like cocaine), but also report feeling a greater sense of openness, appreciation of music and desire to dance, (similar to ecstasy). As well as being legal, it was widely available, and cheap, costing about [†]£10 a gram or £1–2.50 a dose.

The harms and benefits of taking mephedrone

Of the dozens of deaths in 2009 that the media attributed to mephedrone, only two have been confirmed as being directly and solely caused by the drug. One of these was a [†]46-year old man with underlying health problems who repeatedly injected large doses intravenously. Mephedrone was also recorded: as a factor in a handful of other cases; as part of the cocktail in a few mixed-drug deaths; and as having contributed to the mental states of two people who committed suicide. There have been some cases of people with hyponatraemia after taking mephedrone, where low sodium levels lead to swelling in the brain, as happened to Leah Betts when she took ecstasy

Each of these deaths is extremely sad, and anyone would wish they hadn't happened. However, because many people switched to using mephedrone from cocaine, which is a more harmful drug, it may actually have saved lives overall. Statistician Professor Sheila Bird has suggested that the drop in deaths from cocaine, from 95 in the first six months of 2008, to 66 in the first half of 2009, may have been due to this switch, and she calculated that [†]about 40 deaths have been avoided. There was also a [†]drop in soldiers testing positive for cocaine in the army so far fewer were kicked out, so that many careers and lots of taxpayers' money were saved. In addition, the British government gained [†]£600,000 in import tax.

We now know a little about the harms of mephedrone. Users report negative effects such as jaw clenching, nausea, anxiety, insomnia, paranoia and hallucinations, related probably to lack of sleep. Heavy users may well experience insomnia, and there is also the danger of paranoia or even triggering a psychotic episode. Most of these negative effects are relatively mild and short-lived, but some users end up in hospital, usually presenting with a fast and irregular heartbeat, tightness in the chest, agitation, excessive sweating and headaches. Most worryingly, [†]up to 85% of users have reported experiencing cravings for the drug, making it likely that some are using it compulsively and becoming dependent. The desire to redose rapidly seems to be more acute when people snort the powder rather than eating it, which makes sense, as the faster a drug hits the brain, the more addictive it is.

Because use of the drug is so recent, we have very little knowledge about its long-term effects. A lot of people were taking it in Israel for a number of years, and there doesn't seem to have been a large increase in harms as a result. There's now a lot of research taking place around the world into its effects. An Australian survey of ecstasy users found that those also using mephedrone were [†]more likely to have engaged in risky sexual behaviour, which may be related to the fact that it seems to increase sexual drive more than ecstasy.

Why was mephedrone banned?

Louis Wainwright and Nicholas Smith were found dead on March 16th, three weeks before the 2010 UK general election was called. With the dangers of "meow meow" making headlines and an election looming, it was almost inevitable that Home Secretary Alan Johnson would push for mephedrone to be made illegal as soon as possible. The ACMD, who were in the midst of producing a report on cathinones, were asked to speed up the process, and on March 31st published their recommendation that all the synthetic cathinones be placed in Class B. According to one member, [†]the report was only in draft form and still under discussion when the chair rushed off to give Alan Johnson their recommendation in time for him to brief the press.

The period after a general election has been called is known as the "wash up", where legislation that the government wants to push through with the minimum amount of consideration can get fast-tracked into law. In this case all three parties agreed with the amendment to the Misuse of Drugs Act banning the cathinones, so it was debated for an hour and passed without a vote. At such a politically sensitive time, it was highly unlikely that any politician would have stood up and pointed out that at this stage [†]we had almost no evidence (Figure 7.1) that the drug actually caused harm.

The ACMD's report was notable for its lack of hard evidence about mephedrone. Given the lack of formal studies on the psychopharmacology, kinetics, or dynamics of the drug, the Council's knowledge was limited to 25 mephedrone-related presentations at Guy's and St Thomas' Hospital, and the National Addiction Centre's survey of 2000 *Mixmag* readers. The report had been commissioned to look at several different forms of cathinone, but it was mephedrone that was being widely used, and mephedrone that the government wanted to ban, mentioning it by name in the final piece of legislation. Yet Table 7.1, for example, shows the state of our knowledge about its pharmacology as parliament was pushing the bill through.

	Dopamine	Serotonin	Noradrenaline
Amphetamine	•••	•	••••
MDMA	••	•••	•••
Cathinone	•••	••	•••
Methcathinone	•••	•	•••
Methylone	••	•••	••••
Mephedrone	?	?	?

Table 7.1: Actions of selected drugs on different neurotransmitters. This table shows the "relative affinity" between a drug and each of the three neurotransmitters – how effectively the drug targets the dopamine, noradrenaline and serotonin receptors in the brain. •••• is the most effective. • is the least effective. As you can see, the ACMD had no data for mephedrone at all.

Two of my former colleagues quit the ACMD in protest: [†]Eric Carlin said the decision to ban mephedrone was *"unduly based on media and political pressure"*, and [†]Dr Polly Taylor said that she *"did not have trust"* in the way that the government would use the council's advice. Those who stayed were also vocal in their criticism. Criminologist Fiona Measham described the media's portrayal of the unconfirmed deaths as involving [†]*"the usual cycle of exaggeration, distortion, inaccuracy and sensationalism"* we've come to expect in the reporting of recreational drug use. Alan Johnson himself admitted in interview a few months after the election that the [†]media's obsession with the drug sped up the decision to ban it yet he still made the ridiculous assertion that there had been a high-quality scientific review of the evidence: [†]*"The unanimous recommendation to ban the drug made by the scientists, clinicians and other experts on the Advisory Council on the Misuse of Drugs to prevent tragedies in the future was based on painstaking evidence."*

The immediate consequence of the ban was that the price went up. The cost per gram has now quadrupled to [†]about £50, which may have helped to reduce use, although this money is now entirely in the black market, untaxable and being channelled into other sorts of criminal activity. Surprisingly, mephedrone's purity does not seem to have significantly declined, which is probably part of the reason it has stayed so popular since it was criminalised.

The designer drug problem

There are many reasons why mephedrone rose meteorically from little-known pest control agent to household name. In 2009–10 there was definitely a gap in the market for a substitute for cocaine and ecstasy, because at the time these were of exceptionally poor quality. The average purity of cocaine dropped [†]as low as 22% in 2009, and many of the [†]ecstasy pills seized in mid-2010 contained no MDMA at all. ([†]A huge seizure of sassafras oil in Cambodia in June 2008, which could have made 245 million doses of MDMA, was probably responsible for this.) In contrast, before the ban [†]most mephedrone was at least 95% pure.

But even if mephedrone had had quite different effects, the appearance of a new "legal high" was inevitable. Since 2005 we've had GBL, spice and benzylpiperazine (known as BZP) being produced in vast quantities and sold over the internet for a brief period until being banned. This is the designer drug problem: as fast as government can legislate against known drugs, chemists around the world design new compounds specifically to get around the law. This process is speeding up, and the internet is the perfect marketplace for new designer drugs. Mephedrone's appearance on the scene has been specifically [†]linked to the banning of BZP at my recommendation as chair of the ACMD. Perhaps the *Daily Mail* will say the entire episode was my fault!

These drugs are by definition new – variations on existing chemicals that have yet to be classified or controlled. We usually know very little about them, and while they are unlikely to be specifically designed to be harmful (unlike variants entering the illegal drug market, like crack, which was developed to be more addictive) we simply have no idea what their effects will be if they come into widespread use. There is every reason to think that the Chinese factories that were distributing tonnes of mephedrone around the globe in 2010 are already churning out the next legal high.

Alternative approaches

So what can governments do? One approach is to copy the USA, and make analogues of existing controlled substances illegal automatically. This approach is now being suggested by the ACMD, despite the fact that the USA drug enforcement agency has concluded that this is a failed policy, because they find it almost impossible to prosecute under it. And, it would be disastrous for medical research: we know from experience that the use of MDMA as a tool for psychotherapy has been held back for the 40 years since the drug was banned. Already, another cathinone called naphyrone has been made illegal, owing to its chemical similarity to mephedrone, although there is no evidence of widespread use or harm. It was developed as a possible treatment for addiction, and that whole line of research will now suffer as a result of its legal status. And while chemically close to mephedrone, it is also similar to antidepressants such as bupropion, sold under the trade name Wellbutrin. Once you start banning analogues of illegal substances, where exactly do you stop?

What the government have opted for is the introduction of [†]temporary banning orders. These can be brought in as soon as the substance is identified as potentially harmful, and last for 12 months while the ACMD investigates its effects and decides whether it should be included in the Misuse of Drugs Act. Those attempting to import something which has been temporarily banned could receive up to 14 years in prison, but possessing small amounts for personal use would not be a criminal act. As the Drugs Commission has pointed out, the fact that the ACMD's advice doesn't have to be sought before something is banned is a real weakness of this approach, as is the fact that no particular threshold of harm has to be reached before something can be made illegal. This will impact on medical research and industries that work with chemicals, who could see products vital to their work suddenly becoming unavailable without warning.

A different approach, and one I did suggest to the government when I was in the ACMD (though it was predictably rejected) is to follow the example of New Zealand and [†]create a new Class for drugs, Class D. This would be a holding category for new substances, with quality-controlled sales at limited doses restricted to over 18s, and health-education messages on the packaging. People will know what they're taking, and we can monitor use while we work out whether it's something that needs stricter controls. We could combine this with drug testing (cf the Dutch Drug Information and Monitoring System, page 124) and with greater use of amnesty bins in clubs, where visitors are required to discard illicit drugs before entering and security staff put anything they find during searches. With this information we would be in a far stronger position to gather evidence about harms and behaviours than with a simple blanket ban. We wouldn't risk criminalising large numbers of young people for experimenting with new substances, and we would avoid knee-jerk reactions to legislate as fast and as harshly as possible. For most young people the effects of being given a criminal record for drug possession will be much more damaging to their lives than the effects of the drug.

Drugs – without the hot air, David Nutt

The very least we ought to know

Above all, whatever approach a government takes, there is a sensible †minimum amount of data we ought to have before a decision is made about a new drug. The ACMD's report about mephedrone wasn't the only one which was notable for its lack of substantial facts. A few months later, †a Europol report recommended a Europe-wide ban, opening its section on mephedrone with: *"There are no formal pharmacokinetic and pharmacodynamic studies on mephedrone. There are no published formal studies assessing the psychological or behavioural effects of mephedrone in humans. In addition, there are no animal studies on which to base an extrapolation of potential effects."* These are the very organisations that ought to be filling in these gaps in our knowledge so we can make informed decisions about how to reduce harm. Yet rather than wait to gather this evidence, they produced recommendations on the basis of almost nothing.

In response to this, the ISCD has developed the idea of a *minimum dataset* – the very least we should know about a drug before we change its legal status. At a bare minimum, we believe we should have information on:

- Pharmacology. What receptors, transporters and enzymes are relevant to this drug? (Tests should take less than 4 weeks.)
- Basic toxicology. What effects does it have at different doses? How much is an effective dose, and how much is lethal? How does it interact with other drugs? (Tests should take 8 weeks.)
- Human psychopharmacology. What is the subjective experience of users? (An online survey could be done in 16 weeks.)

Ideally, we would also know some other things about the drug. We can establish how addictive it is, and whether it has a withdrawal syndrome, by doing experiments on rodents. These are standard tests which are performed all the time by pharmaceutical companies, are not difficult to set up and run, and should take no more than a month. It would be useful to know the drug's chemistry, whether it dissolves in water, or evaporates at a low enough temperature to be smoked, so we can predict how it's likely to be taken. Equally, the most likely form the drug will be sold in on the street is as a hydrochloride salt, so we should synthesise these and study new drugs in that form.

Another thing we could do to learn more about new drugs as they appear is to set up a †Drugs Information and Monitoring System (DIMS) like the one they have in the Netherlands, which is a fascinating example of applying common sense to drug use. Across the Netherlands there are a number of hospitals where drugs can be tested. Users take their drugs to the centre knowing that they will not be arrested. After the tests they are given information on what the drug is, health and safety advice to help them decide whether to take it or not, and what to do if they get adverse effects. Not only does this offer an opportunity for harm prevention, but also the Dutch authorities get to know exactly what drugs are in circulation and where, and they can catch "bad batches" before they do too much damage. We should set up a similar system in the UK.

Conclusion

There are some important †lessons to be learnt from the mephedrone debacle. The first is that the police shouldn't make public statements or hold press conferences on the basis of hearsay or presumption, and the media should apply some traditional journalistic principles to their coverage of issues around drugs, especially legal highs. Gathering evidence, giving coroners time to undertake proper drug testing, and generally allowing the scientific process to take place before claiming that the drug is harmful, serves the public interest far better than generating hysteria. People understand that much of the reporting on these issues is exaggerated, which is why the media coverage of the supposed harms of mephedrone led to an increase in use. If the media, police, or any other public body wants to be trusted by the public they need to limit themselves to reporting facts, and be seen to do so.

The government and its advisers need to focus on making decisions based on evidence rather than headlines. There needs to be proper research investment into the science of new drugs. Obtaining basic pharmacological facts about mephedrone would have taken at most a few weeks, at little cost, and yet the ACMD's nine-month review didn't even contain these. Having some guidelines on what a report should include, like our minimum dataset, would be a step in the right direction. This would be compatible with temporary banning orders, although I think they are an inadequate response to the radical overhaul of the Misuse of Drugs Act that we need.

Should mephedrone have been banned? The ban may well increase the harms rather than reduce them, as users switch back to more harmful substances like cocaine. An editorial in the *Lancet* shortly after the ban criticised both the government's attitude to the ACMD, and the rushed process to recommend making mephedrone Class B. As they said: [†]"It is too easy and potentially counterproductive to ban each new substance that comes along rather than seek to understand more about young people's motivations and how we can influence them ... Making the drug illegal will also deter crucial research on this drug and other drug-related behaviour, and it will be far more difficult for people with problems to get help."

However, the ban is now in place and there is probably little we can do to change this until the Misuse of Drugs Act is completely restructured, so that it fits the evidence as it should. In the immediate term, we need to properly assess the consequences of the ban to see whether use declines and whether the goal of harm reduction is achieved. This must take into account the harms of criminalising users and monitor any increase in criminal activity associated with dealing and importation; these harms will need to be less than those of the drug itself or the policy will have failed.

A final lesson from this episode is the need to educate people about the dangers of poly drug use, especially mixing other things with alcohol. When new drugs appear, we really don't know how they will interact with others, and mixing them could substantially increase the harms. With alcohol it is particularly important not to combine it with other drugs that suppress breathing, like opiates and GHB/GBL. This is what killed Hester Stewart, who took GBL after she had been drinking, as well as Joslyne Cockburn, Louis Wainwright and Nicholas Smith. If in doubt, *don't drink and drug.*

The original cathinone: khat

[†]Khat is a shrub that grows in East Africa and on the Arab Peninsula. Its leaves have mild stimulant properties when chewed, similar to the leaves of the coca plant that grows in South America. Although the drug is rarely used outside a few cultural and national groups – mostly Somalis, Yemenis and Ethiopians – they've taken the habit with them as they have migrated across the world, creating a small global trade.

The young leaves of the plant contain most cathinone, and are imported from producer countries fresh by air every day wrapped in bundles bound with banana leaves. The first effects are felt after about an hour of chewing, with a typical chewing session lasting 3 to 4 hours, over which time one or two bundles are chewed. The effects are similar to strong coffee – users feel alert and talkative, with sensations of elation and heightened self-esteem; some people say it makes them more imaginative, with a greater capacity to associate ideas. It doesn't have any formal therapeutic uses, but some studies have suggested it may help reduce phobias, and possibly lower cholesterol. For migrant communities, khat chewing is an important social glue that keeps a sense of connection with their countries of origin and helps them share news and resources.

Although we rated khat as one of the least harmful drugs overall, it is still associated with a range of medical and social problems. The practicalities of chewing mean that it's probably impossible to overdose, but there are high levels of oral cancers in khat-consuming countries, and users have an increased risk of heart attacks. There have been cases of hepatitis and cirrhosis in heavy chewers, and about 50% of users develop precancerous white lesions in their mouths. It is known to lower sperm count and can cause constipation, sleep problems and loss of appetite.

Drugs – without the hot air, David Nutt

With many of these health problems, it can be hard to establish if the cathinone itself is the cause. Khat is usually consumed in poorly ventilated "mafreshi" (chewing houses) along with a large number of cigarettes, so much of the increased risk of cancers and heart attacks may actually be due to smoke inhalation. Dangerous pesticides have been detected on the leaves, which people are reluctant to wash off because they believe it reduces the leaves' potency. Users often consume a lot of fizzy drinks as they chew, which may cause tooth decay and diabetes, and young people are now trying to increase the stimulant effect by having caffeine drinks at the same time, which will put more strain on the heart.

Chewing is a very slow method of releasing a drug, which makes it far less addictive than synthetic cathinones like mephedrone. Still, tolerance does develop, and some studies have found up to 40% of users showing signs of dependency. There does seem to be an association between experience of traumatic events, heavy khat use and psychosis, but whether the khat is a trigger or coping mechanism is unclear. It may be that, as with cannabis and schizophrenia, khat relieves some of the symptoms of psychologically vulnerable people, while making others worse. Violence, mood swings and depression are also associated with heavy use.

These behavioural changes can cause social problems for chewers and their families. Heavy users – who are usually men – absenting themselves physically and psychologically for hours at a time can cause family tensions, especially if a significant proportion of their income is being spent on the drug. Since the tobacco-smoking ban, some men have taken to hosting chewing parties in their homes, disrupting time for homework and leaving the women without a social space as it's seen as a single sex activity. Women who do use the drug tend to do so alone, and seem more likely than men to become dependent, possibly because there aren't the same cultural controls around using it socially – just as those who drink at home are more likely to become dependent than those who drink in the pub. Job prospects can be hampered by long hours spent chewing, or being late or absent from work because of lack of sleep. This can be a real problem among marginalised communities who find it difficult to get work anyway.

It's probably partly because khat chewing has not really caught on in Western countries, as much as the fact that it's not very harmful, that has allowed it to avoid legal controls, by and large. Two exceptions are the USA and Canada, which, because they still cling to the belief that banning drugs reduces use, made it illegal some years ago. This led to predictable increases in price, in criminal activity, and even gang deaths, without obvious improvements in public health – a reprise of the situation with alcohol prohibition 70 years earlier. One of the most common issues that UK embassies in the USA and Canada have to deal with now are khat "mules" being arrested at airports. These unfortunate and often innocent people get criminal records, often with imprisonment, and cost the British government a lot of money in dealing with them, just for carrying a leaf that is legal in the UK.

Khat is a source of tension amongst many immigrant communities in the UK, with some seeing it as an important piece of their cultural heritage, and others as a real hindrance to improving their economic situation. Harm reduction measures could include ensuring that dealers wash leaves to get rid of pesticides, providing reliable information about the drug's effects, discouraging simultaneous smoking, and developing treatments for dependence. An outright ban would be disproportionate, and might result in the worst possible perverse consequence – another vulnerable and marginalised social group replacing a relatively harmless drug like khat with a more dangerous one, such as alcohol or amphetamines.

Notes

Page

114　they hadn't taken mephedrone at all• *Teenagers' deaths "not caused by mephedrone"*, BBC news, URL-48, May 28th 2010

114　Joslyne Cockburn• *Teenager's Death Latest Linked to Mephedrone*, Andy Bloxham, URL-49, March 30th 2010

Drugs – without the hot air, David Nutt

115 died from bronchopneumonia caused by a streptococcal A infection• *Police Rule Out 'Legal High' Link To Death*, Lulu Sinclair, URL-50, December 16th 2009

115 ripped off his own scrotum• *Legal drug teen ripped his scrotum off*, Vince Soodin, URL-51, November 26th 2009

115 though this turned out to have been made up• *Mephedrone: the anatomy of a drug media scare*, Nic Fleming, URL-52, April 5th 2010

115 the media through publicising the drug were contributing to its astronomical rise in use• *Virtually a drug scare: Mephedrone and the impact of the Internet on drug news transmission*, AJM Forsyth, International Journal of Drug Policy, 2012. See also URL-166.

116 Israeli scientists working for an insecticide company started experimenting with cathinones• *Mephedrone – scientific background*, ISCD, URL-53, accessed December 10th 2011

116 survey of Tayside schoolchildren and university students in February 2010• *How bubbles blasted its way into Tayside*, Graham Huband, URL-54, May 31st 2010

117 fourth most popular drug amongst clubbers• *Mixmag survey 2009*, Winstock, A. (2010) Results of the 2009/10 Mixmag drug survey. Oral evidence to the ACMD.

117 £10 a gram• *Consideration of the Cathinones*, ACMD, March 31st 2010

117 46-year old man with underlying health problems who repeatedly injected large doses intravenously• npSAD (National Programme on Substance Abuse Deaths) *Drug related deaths in the UK Annual Report*, URL-55, 2009

117 about 40 deaths have been avoided• *Banned drug may have saved lives, not cost them*, Sheila Bird, Statistics Bulletin, URL-56, November 22nd 2010

117 drop in soldiers testing positive for cocaine in the army so far fewer were kicked out• *Mephedrone and cocaine: clues from Army testing*, Sheila Bird and Patrick Mercer, URL-57, accessed December 10th 2011

117 £600,000 in import tax• URL-58, April 8th 2010

118 up to 85% of users have reported experiencing cravings for the drug• *Instability of the ecstasy market and the new kid on the block: mephedrone*, Brunt et al, Journal of Psychopharmacology, September 8th 2010

118 more likely to have engaged in risky sexual behaviour• *Mephedrone use among regular ecstasy consumers in Australia*, Ecstasy and related drug trends Bulletin, URL-59, December 2010

118 the report was only in draft form and still under discussion when the chair rushed off to give Alan Johnson their recommendation in time for him to brief the press• Lancet editorial, URL-60, April 17th 2010

119 we had almost no evidence (Figure 7.1)• *Consideration of the cathinones*, URL-167, ACMD, March 31st, 2010

119 Eric Carlin said the decision to ban mephedrone was *"unduly based on media and political pressure"*• *Government adviser Eric Carlin quits over mephedrone*, BBC News, URL-61, April 2nd 2010

120 Dr Polly Taylor said that she *"did not have trust"*• *Mephedrone to be made Class B drug within week*, BBC News, URL-61, March 29th 2010

120 *"the usual cycle of exaggeration, distortion, inaccuracy and sensationalism"*• *Tweaking, bombing, dabbing and stockpiling: the emergence of mephedrone and the perversity of prohibition*, Measham, F.; Moore, K.; Newcombe, R.; Smith, Z., *Drugs and Alcohol Today* 10 (1), March 12th 2010

120 media's obsession with the drug sped up the decision to ban it• *Addicted to distortion: the media and UK drugs policy*, Jon Silverman, Safer Communities 9 (4), 2010

120 *"The unanimous recommendation to ban the drug made by the scientists, clinicians and other experts on the Advisory Council on the Misuse of Drugs to prevent tragedies in the future was based on painstaking evidence."*• *Decision to outlaw mephedrone drug not connected to teen deaths*, This Is Scunthorpe, URL-62, January 11th 2011

120 about £50• *Mephedrone: still available and twice the price*, Winstock, Mitcheson and Marsden, URL-63, November 6th 2010

120 as low as 22% in 2009• *Miaow Miaow on trial: truth or trumped up charges?*, Nic Fleming, URL-64, March 29th 2010

120 ecstasy pills seized in mid-2010 contained no MDMA at all• *Ecstasy "disappearing" from British clubs*, Jim Reed, URL-65, June 20th 2010

120 A huge seizure of sassafras oil• *World Wired Web*, Mike Power, in *How mephedrone shook the drug trade* issue of *DrugLink*, January/February 2010

120 most mephedrone was at least 95% pure• *Consideration of the Cathinones*, ACMD, March 31st 2010

121 linked to the banning of BZP• *Mephedrone and the ACMD: lessons from BZP and New Zealand's "Class D" experiment?*, Transform, URL-66, March 18th 2010

122 temporary banning orders• *Misuse of Drugs: Temporary Class Drugs*, Home Office, URL-67, August 2011

122 create a new Class for drugs, Class D• *Mephedrone: the Class D solution*, David Nutt, URL-68, March 17th 2010

123 minimum amount of data• *ISCD suggested minimum data set for any new drug that raises concerns about harms*, ISCD, URL-69, accessed December 10th 2011

123 a Europol report• *Joint Report on a new psychoactive substance: 4-methylmethcathinone (mephedrone)*, Europol–EMCDDA, URL-70, March 2010

124 Drugs Information and Monitoring System (DIMS) like the one they have in the Netherlands• *The Drug Information and Monitoring System (DIMS) in the Netherlands: Implementation*, results, and international comparison, Tibor Brunt, Raymond Niesink, Drug Testing and Analysis, 2011

124 lessons to be learnt from the mephedrone debacle• *Hysteria and hubris: lessons on drugs control from the Scunthorpe Two*, David Nutt, URL-71, May 28th 2010

125 "It is too easy and potentially counterproductive to ban each new substance that comes along• *A collapse in integrity of scientific advice in the UK*, Lancet editorial, URL-60, April 17th, 2010

126 Khat is• *Khat (Qat): Assessment of the risk to individuals and communities in the UK*, ACMD, URL-72, December 2005

8 What is addiction? Is there an "addictive personality"?

Using substances from outside the body to change our brain chemistry is something humans have always done, and the psychoactive effects created are similar to the changes we experience when we eat nice food or take exercise. For the majority of people the majority of the time, this doesn't lead to compulsive behaviour – we remain in control, and pretty soon our brains return to their prior state. For a minority, however, drug use leads to drug abuse and addiction, just as a minority of people become addicted to food, gambling or sex. For these people, satisfying their cravings for whatever it is they're addicted to becomes the most powerful source of motivation in their life, overpowering every other need and often leading them to harm themselves and others.

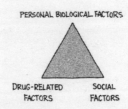

PERSONAL BIOLOGICAL FACTORS

DRUG-RELATED FACTORS   SOCIAL FACTORS

Figure 8.1: The three elements that affect whether a person becomes addicted to a particular drug.

There are three elements that affect whether a person becomes addicted to a particular drug (Figure 8.1):

1. *Drug-related factors* include how the drug reaches the brain, and what it does when it gets there. Tolerance and   withdrawal also affect its addictiveness.

2. *Social factors* include the availability and acceptability of using the drug, the prevalence of advertising, how the drug makes groups behave, and the economic and social costs.
3. *Personal and biological factors* are factors such as age, gender and genetics.

In this chapter we look at the mechanisms of addiction, tolerance and withdrawal, and why certain people seem to have "addictive personalities". (Chapter 4 has already examined some of the drug-related factors, which we explore in more detail in chapter 10, and we cover the social factors in chapter 11.)

Addiction in history

Our understanding of addiction has increased as more drugs have become available, and as their role in society has changed. Until the 19th century, heavy drinking or use of other drugs wasn't seen as a special category of behaviour, but as a sin of excess, similar to overeating – gluttony was a problem because you were eating *too much*, not because food itself was a bad thing. Although excessive use of drugs was seen as problematic, the majority of people usually didn't have access to enough potent substances to have that problem. An exception was the †Gin Craze, of the 18th century. Technological advances and several years of good harvests led to a fall in the price of food, giving the urban poor in London discretionary income for the first time, which they started to spend on the powerful liquor that was being made from the grain surplus. Alcohol harms increased substantially, especially amongst the more vulnerable members of society. This changed the general perception of alcohol, and eventually led to the formation of the Temperance Movement, which recognised that there was something particular about alcoholic beverages that led to patterns of dangerous and compulsive use. What really ended the Craze, however, was a series of bad harvests, which pushed up the price of food again and reduced the availability of gin.

As purer and more powerful substances became available at the end of the 19th century, drugs started to be seen as a special sort of social menace, and our understanding of addiction started to be seen in psychological terms. Someone with an "addictive personality" was considerd morally weak, unable to resist the temptation posed by drugs, unlike good law-abiding citizens. Now that there was widespread access to drugs, it became clear that there was some kind of [†] relationship between being marginalised from society and drug addiction. The fact that groups like Native Americans, Australian aborigines, gay people and poor people seemed to be more likely to become addicts was seen as confirming the moral basis for their place in the social order. Willpower alone was thought to be enough to give up drugs, possibly accompanied by therapy to uncover the psychological reasons for becoming addicted. Therapists were trained in Freudian psychoanalysis, and would search for underlying causes of addiction such as repressed childhood memories or the fear of taking on the responsibilities of adulthood.

It's interesting that throughout this period the habitual use of one of the most common and harmful drugs of all – tobacco – wasn't even recognised as an addiction. The fact that most politicians and doctors (including Freud) were hooked on it themselves must have contributed to this blind spot!

In the second half of the twentieth century, developments in our understanding of how the brain works challenged this approach. The discovery of chemicals in the brain that work in similar ways to common drugs of abuse, and receptors apparently designed to respond to them, led to addiction being analysed in biological rather than psychological terms. We now understand that repeated use of a drug can cause physical changes to our brains, resulting in a kind of "brain disease", in the same way that strain on the heart can lead to heart disease. Neuroimaging techniques in the last 15 years have allowed us to see these changes for the first time, confirming that these changes are physical and to an extent irreversible. (See box *How does neuroimaging work?* on page 150.)

As with any other sort of disease, individuals are at risk of addiction to different degrees depending on their genes, background and environment. If people in marginalised groups are more likely to become addicts, this is because of the stress caused by their position in society, not because being a member of that particular group makes them weak and immoral. An "addictive personality" is now understood to describe someone who is particularly vulnerable to this disease, not someone lacking in willpower. Addiction is largely preventable and treatable, just as diabetes is, but for some people the make-up of their brain or the circumstances of their life make addiction almost inevitable, and blaming them for their vulnerability is unfair. To put it another way: †when a highly educated, high-status man like David Cameron, who is protected from drug abuse by numerous factors in his life (such as being born to a rich family and going to a top school and university) uses cannabis and doesn't get addicted, this isn't because he's morally superior to someone else who does become addicted. The same is true for †President Obama, who has admitted to cocaine use before he came to office.

Some recent work has identified the neurological similarities between drug addictions and other types of behavioural addiction, such as compulsive eating or gambling, which seem to involve the same psychological and biological mechanisms in the brain. Researchers such as Jim Orford have suggested †we ought to think of drug addiction as a special form of behavioural addiction, which can occur with any (initially) pleasurable activity, from shopping to exercise. In some ways, this takes us full circle, to a pre-19th century model of excessive behaviour – drugs do have some special qualities, but the mechanisms by which they can become the most powerful drives in people's lives are similar to those involved in other pleasurable and repeated activities. These mechanisms are both psychological and biological, and are central to how our brains work.

The brain mechanisms of addiction

Addiction involves both the pleasure chemicals in the brain, and the processes by which we learn repeated behaviours. This process is very complicated, involving many mechanisms and different neurotransmitters. Figure 8.2 shows some of the different elements involved. On the left, we can see the positive elements of a drug experience – it might create pleasure, reduce suffering, lay down powerful memories or reveal a new perspective that seems particularly meaningful.

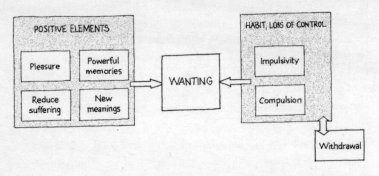

Figure 8.2: The various elements of addiction.

On the right, are the elements that drive us back to repeat the experience. Being impulsive – thinking primarily about short-term effects rather than long-term consequences – or generally prone to repetitious, compulsive behaviour, can lead to a lack of control which makes it especially difficult to resist the desire to re-experience the positive elements of the drug. Alongside these elements of habit are the unpleasant effects of withdrawal, which are at best uncomfortable and at worst life-threatening. The "pull" factors on the left, combined with the "push" factors on the right, create an overwhelming sense of wanting, which can overpower someone's conscious knowledge of the damage that a drug might do to them.

Figure 8.3 shows how [†]different neurotransmitters are believed to be involved in these "push" and "pull" factors. Dopamine is involved in drive and desire and perhaps reward; endorphins give peace and pleasure, reduce suffering, and numb pain; GABA and glutamate regulate memory; serotonin may be involved in attributing meaning to experience. Noradrenaline seems to be related to impulsivity and compulsivity, which is why amphetamines can help people with attention disorders – because stimulants reduce impulsivity.

Dopamine seems to play a key part in addiction. It is released in special

Drugs – without the hot air, David Nutt

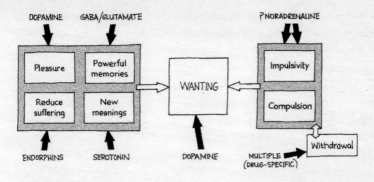

Figure 8.3: The neurotransmitters that regulate the elements of addiction.

brain regions when we feel a sense of reward and achievement, helping us to learn what we did to feel good so we know to repeat the activity in the future. Neuroimaging has allowed us to see dopamine being released when people take cocaine and other stimulants and also when we succeed at activities such as playing video games. Addiction to video gaming is becoming increasingly common, especially as the internet makes 24-hour play possible. (An extreme example of this was the [†]Korean couple who let their baby starve to death while they played a computer game that involved rearing a virtual child.)

We now know that having an unusually low number of dopamine receptors seems to predispose people to experiencing excessive pleasure when they use stimulants. This excessive response is thought to start happening in the reward centre of the brain – the nucleus accumbens – but over weeks or months of use moves into other areas where habits are laid down, a shift from voluntary (choice-use) to involuntary (habit-use). Addiction can be seen as a loss of control over what starts out as a voluntary behaviour.

This loss of control has two factors. A drug can enhance the "push" factors, creating an overwhelming desire to do something, or it can reduce our ability to resist behaviours, even if we know they will have negative consequences. Most often it's a combination of both. Over time, this can lead to an inability to resist cravings which a non-addict has no difficulty in overcoming. This explains a common complaint of addicts that they don't want to continue with their addictions and don't enjoy them anymore, but can't stop because taking the drug has become a kind of involuntary reflex.

Addiction is particularly common among people with lower numbers of dopamine receptors, and this is true even for drugs which don't directly release dopamine themselves. Alcohol primarily stimulates the GABA receptors, for example, but studies of alcoholics and their families have found that [†]alcoholics have fewer dopamine receptors than their non-alcoholic relatives. Increasing the number of dopamine receptors also reduces alcohol intake. In [†]tests on rats that have been made addicted to alcohol, injecting them with a virus that makes more dopamine receptors results in the rats drinking less.

The issue of the number of dopamine receptors an individual has is complicated, however, because although this is partly genetically determined, the number can vary according to our environment as well. Tests with rhesus monkeys, who have similar social patterns to humans, have found that [†]high-status monkeys have more dopamine receptors than low-status monkeys, and lower-status ones take more cocaine and alcohol when exposed to these drugs. Even more interestingly, the number of receptors can change over time in response to social experiences. When the dominance is reversed, the number of receptors in the monkey that was formerly lower status goes up, and the amount of cocaine it takes goes down.

A further complication is that using some drugs, particularly stimulants such as crack and methamphetamine, reduces the number of dopamine receptors in the brain. This results in a vicious cycle where an addict's ability to feel pleasure or reward from any other activity diminishes the more they take the drug (Figure 8.4).

If dopamine is involved in motivation and drive, it's the brain's natural opiates (endorphins, enkephalins and dynorphins) that give us the sensation of reward. When these chemical messengers are released they make you feel happy and reduce pain; they also play an important role in mother/child bonding. Heroin and other opiates primarily interact

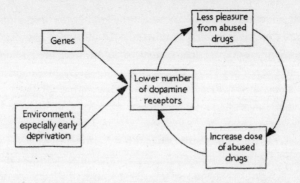

Figure 8.4: How dopamine may be involved in the vicious cycle of drug abuse.

with this system, changing the receptors in a way similar to how stimulants change dopamine receptors. This means that heroin addicts often feel miserable even when they are "clean". We are learning that many other drugs that mainly work on other types of receptors also interact with endorphin receptors. Alcohol seems to release endorphins, which is why some new treatments for alcohol dependence involve using drugs that block these receptors, stopping alcohol-induced pleasure or craving. There's some evidence that endorphins are also involved in our development of liking for tobacco and stimulants. Some recent work from my research group has shown that [†]amphetamine releases endorphins, which may help us to develop new treatments for addiction to this kind of stimulant.

What is tolerance and why does it occur?

Tolerance occurs when repeatedly doing something changes the way we react to it. When we take drugs, the brain usually responds to the overstimulation that the drugs cause, by desensitising the target receptors – each hit creates less of a high so you need to take successively larger doses to achieve the same effect. The more frequently you take a drug, the more quickly tolerance builds up, because your brain has less time between doses to readjust. For example, [†]if you use ketamine about once a month, an effective dose could be as little as 20 mg, whereas if you use it daily you might eventually need to take 200 mg to feel any effect at all. The most extreme form of tolerance happens during binges, when someone keeps themselves in a constant state of intoxication for a prolonged period, sometimes as long as a couple of days. Figure 8.5 shows a graph of brain activity during a cocaine binge:

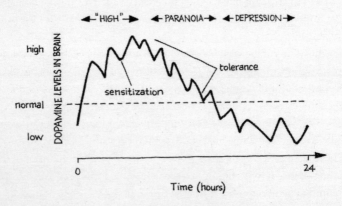

Figure 8.5: Bingeing on cocaine leads to increased tolerance in a very short space of time.

Tolerance occurs to protect us from the risk of overdose. Alcoholics can consume several times the volume of alcohol that would put non-alcoholics into a coma. A recent study found that one in eight prisoners overdose on heroin or methadone within two weeks of being released. Having stopped or reduced their intake in prison, their tolerance is reset, so if they take what was their usual dose prior to going to jail their brain can't cope and they overdose. About 500 people a year die as a result of this.

Sometimes people can develop "reverse tolerance", where repeated use leads to extreme sensitisation instead of the normal reduced sensitivity. Some cocaine users, for example, can suddenly find themselves acutely sensitive to its effects. This is dangerous, because it can cause effects such as seizures. However, it might possibly have some therapeutic benefits: some of my earliest research was on the possibility of creat-

Drugs – without the hot air, David Nutt

ing an anti-depressant effect by using sensitisation to cocaine to increase dopamine function in the brain. (The experiments weren't very successful – we could show it happened but couldn't identify a mechanism or understand why!)

Psychedelics create an interesting form of tolerance – a huge and sudden decrease in effects that lasts about a week, so that taking LSD straight after your last trip will have almost no effect at all. This makes bingeing almost impossible, and is one of the reasons why psychedelics are very rarely abused.

†Sensitisation can be seen in behavioural addictions such as gambling. People respond to "near wins" (getting three out of four matches on a fruit machine, for example) with a sense of reward almost as good as if they'd actually won something. This encourages them to continue playing, as they're getting some of the high they want even though they're actually losing. Fruit machines and scratch-card lotteries are often designed to ensure a higher-than-chance frequency of near misses – the sensation of nearly winning can be created when a fruit machine shows two winning symbols and a third just below or above it, for example.

Withdrawal and craving

Just as the brain tries to reduce drug-induced overstimulation by building up tolerance, when users stop taking the drug the brain suddenly has to adapt again. This is called withdrawal, and can be extremely unpleasant or even life-threatening. Physical withdrawal usually consists of the opposite effects of the drug: being high on amphetamine makes you feel energised, while amphetamine withdrawal makes you feel lethargic; taking heroin makes you relaxed and pain-free, while in withdrawal, users are jittery and acutely sensitive to pain; alcohol relaxes people and calms their brains, whereas in withdrawal the brain is hyper-excitable and users are anxious and can even have fits.

As well as physical symptoms there are psychological effects. Most withdrawing addicts suffer from low dopamine levels, creating *anhedonia* (a form of depression that makes them unable to feel pleasure). This can last for weeks, months or even years, creating powerful cravings for the drug, and is usually the strongest force driving addicts to relapse. Jim Orford has suggested that a lot of [†]addiction starts as pleasure seeking, but when withdrawal kicks in, the main drive becomes reducing the suffering of withdrawal. This is particularly true for most smokers: tobacco is usually unpleasant to start with, but once someone is addicted withdrawal is even more unpleasant so relieving that discomfort is experienced as pleasurable (Figure 8.6).

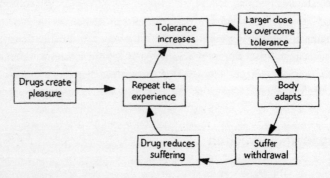

Figure 8.6: Drug abuse starts as pleasure-seeking but ends up as avoiding withdrawal.

There will usually be both physical and psychological symptoms in any withdrawal, and it can be hard to distinguish between the two because expectation plays such an important role in our experiences of drugs. Many regular drug users will feel very attached to the process of preparing and consuming their substance of choice and will crave this context almost as much as the drug itself. Feeling anxious or having trouble sleeping after stopping might be a psychological or psychosomatic response to this sense of loss, rather than a purely physical response. An example of how we can distinguish between physical and psychological symptoms is when cannabis users are given rimonabant, which blocks the effects of the drug on cannabis receptors. The users continue to smoke cannabis, thus satisfying their psychological cravings for it, but don't experience any psychoactive effects. What these studies have shown is that even under these circumstances cannabis users will

Drugs – without the hot air, David Nutt

experience withdrawal symptoms, proving that cannabis has a physical withdrawal syndrome.

Physical withdrawal can be very unpleasant and even life-threatening, but it is relatively short-lived compared with psychological symptoms, which can remain powerful even years after the addict last took the drug. Indeed, it's usually the psychological cravings that drive addicts to relapse long after the purely physical symptoms have passed. However, understanding physical withdrawal does have important implications for treatment, because if these short-term symptoms can be controlled with pharmacological substitutes it makes it much easier to help people to regulate their use in preparation for stopping altogether. In this sense, drug addictions may be easier to treat than other behavioural addictions, where we don't yet have equivalent treatments to help them through the crucial early stages of quitting.

Diagnosing addiction

Most of us will know somebody who drinks ten cups of tea a day, takes sleeping pills every night, or consumes an unhealthy amount of alcohol, but we don't call these people "addicts". So when exactly does drug use become addiction? There's a lot of confusion around the meaning of the word, and it has a lot of negative connotations, which is why when the medical model of addiction was being developed around 50 years ago, groups such as the World Health Organization started talking about a "drug dependence syndrome" instead. The problem is that this term often gets confused with physical dependence (defined as experiencing withdrawal on stopping), but physical dependence in itself isn't sufficient for a diagnosis of "drug dependence". I think the word "addiction" is still useful to refer to a state of repeated drug use characterised by a strong, sometimes overwhelming, desire to take it, despite the fact that it's causing significant difficulties.

Addiction is really about experiencing cravings and losing control over your actions, not just physical tolerance and withdrawal. Although all these often do go hand-in-hand, if the psychological cravings are mild or non-existent we wouldn't call someone an addict. Most of us go into caffeine withdrawal overnight, for example, and some people can experience headaches and lethargy as a result, but very few would find it psychologically traumatic if wasn't available for a while. (There is more about this distinction in chapter 12.)

According to the WHO International Classification of Diseases, a medical diagnosis of "drug dependence syndrome", (or "addiction" as I'll continue to refer to it here) is given when three or more of the following criteria have been present at the same time in the last year:

- Feeling a strong desire or compulsion to take the substance.
- Difficulties in controlling how much you take and how often, and finding yourself unable to stop.
- Physical withdrawal symptoms.
- Signs of tolerance and having to increase your dosage.
- Neglecting other pleasures or interests; spending large amounts of time intoxicated or recovering from the drug.
- Continuing to take the substance even when it is obviously doing you harm.

In practice, diagnosing addiction is a question of motivation. Once somebody's experience of pleasure has become inextricably tied up with the drug, using it can become the most important thing in their lives. This can overwhelm even the most powerful of human emotions such as love for friends and family. Some addicts, particularly women, manage to curb their behaviour when they have children, but for many users even that isn't enough to break the cycle of substance abuse.

It is often difficult for people who have not been addicted, or don't know any addicts, to understand how powerful the motivation for a drug can be. Perhaps the best analogy is being in love. When people fall in love, this state often dominates their lives to the exclusion of all other considerations. They'll go to enormous lengths to be near the person they're in love with, experience withdrawal when they're parted and get intense pleasure when re-united. It may even be that the brain mechanisms of love and addiction share a common process; on a chemical level, endorphins are the most likely neurotransmitters to be involved.

Drugs – without the hot air, David Nutt

The exact form that addiction takes depends on the substance involved and the social context. What we think of as classic drug-seeking behaviours are largely based on people addicted to heroin and crack: committing crimes or engaging in prostitution to buy drugs, stealing from family and friends, lying about drug use, neglecting their children and spending all their time either intoxicated or looking for drugs. Of course, this becomes a vicious cycle: as family and friends stop trusting them, they lose their homes and jobs, go in and out of prison, their children go into care, their lives become more and more miserable and the only thing that can relieve their suffering is the drug.

Some of these negative behaviours are the result of heroin and crack being illegal, and can be reduced by administering the drug (or pharmacological substitutes) in medical settings. If they didn't need to steal to fund their habits, for example, heroin and crack addicts would be less likely to have their lives ruined by being sent to prison.

Tobacco addiction, on the other hand, takes quite a different form. Because it is freely available and each hit is relatively cheap, we don't see "tobacco fiends" committing crimes to feed their habit, and because its intoxication effect is very mild it rarely disrupts people's ability to continue with normal life. What we do see is people making repeated, unsuccessful attempts to quit, experiencing irresistible cravings for the drug even if they haven't taken it for months or years, and continuing to smoke even when suffering serious health consequences, such as lung problems or heart disease.

Is there an "addictive personality"?

Most people use drugs of some form, have sex and take exercise, and everybody eats and shops. A small minority, however, can become addicted to these behaviours, until their need to engage in them overpowers every other motivation in their lives. There are a variety of personal biological factors that make someone predisposed to addiction. Some of these are specific to particular substances, and others are common across all behavioural addictions.

We know of a number of traits that make people vulnerable to specific drugs. There is a genetic component to alcoholism, for example, which has been proved by [†]Danish studies that have shown that the sons of alcoholic fathers have the same elevated risk of developing alcoholism whether they stay with their natural father or are adopted by non-drinkers. There are almost certainly hereditary elements to addictions to other drugs as well. Our genes can determine how quickly we metabolise drugs; this is a consideration in addiction, because the faster we process a drug the more severe our withdrawal reaction will be. [†]The enzyme that clears nicotine from the body has two versions, one which results in a high metabolism and the other in a low metabolism; in studies of withdrawal in smokers, the faster nicotine leaves the body the more likely the person is to relapse when they try to stop.

There are variations on endorphin and GABA receptors which can make people more or less sensitive to certain drugs. Being more sensitive may make you more vulnerable to addiction, because the drug will have a more powerful effect. Conversely, [†]male children of male alcoholics have alterations in GABA receptors that make them *less* sensitive to alcohol so they can consume more than their friends from the first day they start drinking. This makes them drink more, and so become dependent more rapidly. The number of receptors someone has also plays a role. Having low numbers of dopamine receptors, for example, is associated with alcoholism and cocaine use. [†]High opioid receptor levels in the brain also predict drug use and craving for opiates, and possibly for alcohol as well.

Other traits that can affect vulnerability to addiction are environment- and gender-related:

- The conditions someone has experienced in the womb: [†]if mothers use drugs while pregnant, their children may be more likely to become addicted to those same drugs in later life.
- Environmental effects such as trauma and deprivation strongly predict opiate use, especially if experienced in early life.
- Although most addicts are male, drugs usually have more of an effect on women, because women are smaller and have a higher

Drugs – without the hot air, David Nutt

proportion of body fat (and fat doesn't absorb most drugs). The menstrual cycle produces hormones (neurosteroids) that act in the brain and affect the actions of alcohol and other drugs.

In addition to the above features that make people likely to abuse specific drugs, there are general traits that make people more vulnerable to all kinds of addictive and compulsive behaviour. These include:

- Impulsivity. A tendency to act without thought for the long-term consequences of your actions can make you more likely to take drugs and become addicted. On the other hand, stimulants make people less impulsive, and some people take them partly as self-medication for their impulsivity.
- Compulsivity. Compulsive people are less likely to start taking drugs as they are more anxious about negative effects, but find it harder to stop once they started.
- Anxiety and depression. Many people use drugs to get relief from these feelings (which are also associated with low social status, trauma and deprivation).
- Adolescent use. Adolescence is a time when we are particularly vulnerable to forming habits, so starting young may make us more prone to becoming addicted.
- Gender. Men tend to be more sensation-seeking, and there are also social factors around loss of control which make men more likely to become addicts than women.

Protective factors – why some people *don't* get addicted to drugs

There are many reasons why people might be *less* prone to addictive behaviours. The key factors that seem to protect people from drug abuse include:

- Health concerns. Fear of drugs' negative consequences (which may or may not be in proportion to the actual risk), can protect against addiction.
- Regular testing. People who do a lot of sport or are in the army, where drug-testing is common, are often more motivated by their desire to continue with their job or hobby than by their desire to take drugs.
- Bad experiences, especially initial ones. Drugs are inherently unpredictable, and a proportion of people have a bad time when they take them. Negative first experiences tend to stop people from repeating them. A genetic variant that protects against smoking appears to make nicotine more unpleasant when first used.
- Just not liking them. People with lots of dopamine receptors experience less pleasure from cocaine than those with fewer dopamine receptors, and some genetic variants can stop some drugs being pleasurable. For example, the ALDH2 enzyme makes alcohol unpleasant.
- Well-balanced moods. Just as being prone to depression and anxiety makes you more likely to abuse drugs, having well-balanced moods is protective.
- Pledging abstinence. Making public declarations of abstinence, as part of a religious or social group, can create strong social motivations to stay away from drugs.

It is important to maintain a distinction between using drugs and being vulnerable to addiction: many people who don't use drugs at all would be likely to become addicted if they did use them!

Drugs – without the hot air, David Nutt

Conclusion

Humans are natural pleasure-seekers, and pleasure is an essential part of how we learn – it's normal and natural, and usually carries low risk of harm. Yet a minority of people develop behavioural addictions to pleasurable experiences, and these addictions can lead to profoundly miserable lives. Drug addictions are among the most common behavioural addictions because the effects of drugs are usually so much greater than the effects of natural neurotransmitters released from other activities. Some people, however, can experience extreme rushes from activities such as gambling or eating, and can end up engaging in an activity compulsively even though it is harming them and others around them.

Addictions to drugs (as opposed to other activities) do have some distinctive features, such as physical withdrawal symptoms which can drive users back to the drug even if they no longer experience it as pleasurable. Because different drugs target different sets of neurotransmitters very efficiently, they can be appealing to people with certain sorts of brain chemistry. (For example, part of the genetic component of alcoholism seems to be a tendency to have fewer GABA receptors in the brain, so that alcohol relieves the person's near-constant state of anxiety.) These people may find that they struggle to control their use of one particular drug, but that they aren't attracted to other forms of compulsive behaviour. There is growing evidence that alterations in endorphins and their receptors are a risk factor for   heroin, alcohol and cocaine addiction.

Other people find that they get hooked in succession on different activities, (drug-taking or other behaviours). Often they'll "cure" themselves of one addiction simply by replacing it with another. For example, drug users often switch to overeating or exercise, and many young heroin addicts move on to alcohol in their thirties. This is perhaps the closest thing to what you could call an "addictive personality", with common traits being compulsivity, early deprivation, experience of trauma, and low numbers of dopamine receptors. In general, however, it's probably more accurate to talk about "vulnerable personalities" – a range of different environmental and genetic factors which make people more susceptible to addictions.

All of this is important because minimising the harms done by drugs necessarily involves avoiding and treating addiction. In the next chapter, we'll look at whether addiction can be cured, and the most common and effective treatments in use today. As with any other public-health problem, identifying risk factors, in order that people can make informed decisions about what they choose to do, is an essential part of reducing harm. Unravelling the complex factors that drive addiction, and helping people to stay in control of their own behaviour, requires improving our understanding of these risk factors.

How does neuroimaging work?

In the last fifteen years, we've developed new techniques ([†]"neuroimaging") that allow us to take pictures of the brain in action. These have vastly improved our understanding of how the brain is made up and how it works. However, interpreting the images produced is often difficult, partly because there's a lot of variation between individuals, and partly because drug users rarely use just a single drug (making it hard to associate a particular brain activity to a specific drug). At the moment imaging can only show us correlations and say little about causality.

There are two main types of imaging techniques. The first is *positron emission tomography* (*PET*). We can use a radioactive isotope as a "tracer" by attaching it to a substance (such as glucose or a drug), that we know behaves in a certain way in the brain. When injected into the bloodstream the molecules of the glucose or drug are carried into the brain. The isotope has a very short half-life (ie it decays quickly). When an atom of the isotope decays, it emits a positron, which is the same as an electron but has the opposite charge. When the emitted positron collides with an electron, the two annihilate one another and emit energy. Because there are many free electrons in the body, the collision usually occurs less than 1mm from the decaying isotope, ie very close to where the injected substance accumulated in the brain, so if we can pin-point where the collision occurred, we can see where the substance was within the brain. The energy emitted from the collision is seen as two gamma rays radiating at 180 degrees to one another, which can be detected some distance outside the head by the †PET camera. Samples are taken over a period of about an hour; the information about the energy of the gamma rays and whereabouts in the camera they were detected is then processed by a computer to produce an image called a *PET scan* (eg Figure 8.7 on page 152). Here's an example of how PET is used: we know that the chemical flumazenil binds to GABA receptors, so by doing a PET scan on someone who has been injected with a flumazenil tracer we can identify where GABA receptors lie and how many there are in a particular area.

The second technique is *magnetic resonance imaging* (*MRI*). This does not use any radioactive material; instead, it relies on the fact that the body is mainly composed of water. When the body is placed in a strong magnetic field with a constant gradient, the hydrogen ions in the water align themselves along the lines of magnetic force, much like iron filings around a magnet. If we then apply a pulse of energy in the form of a very short blast of radio waves at a particular frequency, the hydrogen ions flip out of their preferred alignment. When the pulse of radio waves ends, the atoms gradually drift back ("relax") to their original position, giving out energy again as radio waves of different frequencies. These radio signals can be detected and the information converted into spatial images. Different tissues relax at different rates, giving very high delineation between the different parts of the anatomy that comprise the image.

Functional MRI (*fMRI*) is a refinement of MRI, and relies on the fact that blood is a magnetic fluid (because of the iron in haemoglobin). Increased metabolism is indicated by increased blood supply and vice versa, so that the parts of the brain that are working "light up" on the image, letting us see which parts of the brain react to different stimuli. FMRI can also be used to explore the parts of the brain involved in internally-generated experiences such as moods, thoughts and memories, including those of addiction such as craving.

Neuroimaging techniques have played a central role in the development of our understanding of addiction. They have enabled us to confirm the role of dopamine in many addictions, although conversely they have also revealed that opiate addiction may not really involve dopamine at all. We've been able to study the parts of the brain involved in craving, by giving cues (such as personalised auditory memories of drug taking) and looking at brain activity. For example, Figure 8.7 shows the distribution of GABA-A receptors in the brain, which is where alcohol takes its effect. However, some drugs are difficult to study with neuroimaging, because we don't have reliable tracers – for example we have yet to find *good* glutamate tracers.

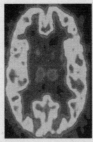

Figure 8.7: The distribution in the brain of GABA-A receptors, which are where alcohol acts.

Currently, neuroimaging is primarily used only in research, in order to improve our understanding of brain mechanisms, evaluate treatments of addiction and discover the reasons behind relapse. It's possible that in the future people will try to use neuroimaging for legal purposes, perhaps to establish diminished responsibility on the basis of the biological formation of a defendant's brain. For now, the imaging techniques show only *correlations* between some aspect of a person's behaviour and the activity of certain parts of the brain; imaging says little about the *causes* of particular behaviours. I think it's unlikely that we'll ever reach that level of sophistication and understanding from snapshot images like those we currently obtain, but it's important that we are prepared for the legal and ethical implications if we do.

Notes

Page

133 Gin Craze, of the 18th century• *Alcohol: First Report of Session 2009–10*, House of Commons Health Committee, December 10th 2009

134 relationship between being marginalised from society and drug addiction• *The Stigma of Substance Abuse: a Review of the Literature*, Centre for Addiction and Mental Health, URL-73, August 18th 1999

135 when a highly educated, high-status man like David Cameron• *Cameron – the rise of the new conservative*, Francis Elliott, Fourth Estate, 2007. See also URL-174, *Cameron admits: I used dope at Eton*, the *Guardian*, February 11, 2007

135 President Obama, who has admitted to cocaine use before he came to office.• For sources see Wikipedia, URL-31.

135 we ought to think of drug addiction as a special form of behavioural addiction• *Problem Gambling and Other Behavioural Addictions*, Jim Orford, in *Drugs and the Future: Brain Science, Addiction and Society*, David Nutt et al, Elsevier, 2007

136 different neurotransmitters are believed to be involved in these "push" and "pull" factors• Which neurotransmitters are involved is still a subject of research.

137 Korean couple who let their baby starve to death• *Girl starved to death while parents raised virtual child in online game*, URL-168, the *Guardian*, March 5th, 2010

138 alcoholics have fewer dopamine receptors than their non-alcoholic relatives• *Overexpression of dopamine D2 receptors reduces alcohol self-administration*, Panayotis K Thanos, Nora D Volkow, et al, Journal of Neurochemistry (78), 2001

138 tests on rats that have been made addicted to alcohol• As above.

138 high-status monkeys have more dopamine receptors than low-status monkeys• *Characterising organism x environment interactions in non-human primate models of addiction: PET imaging studies of D2 receptors*, Michael Nader et al, in The Neurobiology of Addiction, Oxford University Press, 2010

139 amphetamine releases endorphins• *Stimulation of endorphin neurotransmission in the nucleus accumbens by ethanol, cocaine, and amphetamine*, Foster Olive et al, Journal of Neuroscience 21 (1), 2001

139 if you use ketamine about once a month, an effective dose could be as little as 20 mg, whereas if you use it daily you might eventually need to take 200 mg to feel any effect at all• *Ketamine: a scientific review*, Celia Morgan and Valeria Curran, ISCD, September 15th 2010

141 Sensitisation can be seen in behavioural addictions such as gambling• *Problem Gambling and Other Behavioural Addictions*, Jim Orford, in *Drugs and the Future: Brain Science, Addiction and Society*, Nutt et al, Elsevier, 2007

142 addiction starts as pleasure seeking, but when withdrawal kicks in, the main drive becomes reducing the suffering of withdrawal• *Problem Gambling and Other Behavioural Addictions*, Jim Orford, in *Drugs and the Future: Brain Science, Addiction and Society*, David Nutt et al, Elsevier, 2007

146 Danish studies that have shown that the sons of alcoholic fathers• *The Danish longitudinal study of alcoholism 1978–2008*, Joachim Knop, Danish Medical Bulletin, (58) 8, 2011

146 The enzyme that clears nicotine from the body has two versions• *Genetic variability in CYP2A6 and the pharmacokinetics of nicotine*, JC Mwenifumbo and RF Tyndale, *Pharmacogenomics* 8(10), October 2007

146 male children of male alcoholics have alterations in GABA receptors that make them *less* sensitive to alcohol• *Reactions to Alcohol in Sons of Alcoholics and Controls*, Marc Schuckit, Alcoholism: Clinical and Experimental Research 12, 1988

146 High opioid receptor levels in the brain also predict drug use and craving for opiates• *Brain opioid receptor binding in early abstinence from opioid dependence*, Tim Williams et al, British Journal of Psychiatry (191), 2007

146 if mothers use drugs while pregnant, their children may be more likely to become addicted to those same drugs in later life• *Drugs and the Future: Brain Science, Addiction and Society*, David Nutt et al, Elsevier, 2007

150 "neuroimaging"• *Brain imaging in addiction*, David Nutt, Anne Lingford-Hughes and Liam Nestor in *Addiction Neuroethics*, Elsevier, 2012

151 PET camera• which is in fact a "scintillation counter".

9 Can addiction be cured?

Introduction

The previous chapter looked at the concept of addiction, and examined the risk factors that give some people more "addictive personalities" than others. This chapter examines the treatment of addiction, including psychological treatments such as cognitive behavioural therapy, and pharmacological substitutes such as methadone. We also look at ways to evaluate how successful they are, and whether or not addiction can be prevented or "cured".

Case study 1: Tony Adams and alcohol

In the early 1990s, [†]Tony Adams was one of the Premier League's most popular footballers, going from strength to strength on the pitch. Off it, he was battling a serious addiction to alcohol, which landed him in prison for drink-driving, and led to the breakdown of his marriage and his eventual retirement from the game. He hit rock bottom after he went on a 7-week drinking binge following Euro '96, and finally sought help; he credits Alcoholics Anonymous with helping him stay off the booze, and he has now been abstinent for nearly a decade and a half. In an effort to learn to feel pleasure from other activities, he started to educate himself, took up the piano and developed an interest in the arts. He has spoken publicly about his alcoholism, primarily in his autobiography *Addicted*, and has set up a rehabilitation clinic for sportsmen and women with substance-abuse problems.

Case study 2: Pete Doherty, heroin and crack

Pete Doherty, the former singer of the Libertines and Babyshambles, has been engaged in [†]a very public battle with heroin and crack addiction for over a decade. Despite the seriously-harmful consequences his addiction has had on his life, and the knowledge that it will probably kill him, he can't seem to find an effective treatment. He has spent time in jail for stealing from a former band-mate, for drink driving, and for possession of various drugs (most commonly heroin), and at the time of writing is in prison for possession of cocaine. Because of the intense media interest in his drug use, his repeated trips to rehab have been widely publicised, as have his frequent relapses. At Doherty's most recent court appearance his solicitor said "he takes no pleasure in his addiction. It's one thing, he said publicly, he would not wish upon his worst enemy. He is acutely aware of the agonising nature of addiction".

Case study 3: Amy Winehouse

Much like Pete Doherty, singer Amy Winehouse combined a highly successful music career with chronic relapsing addictions to a number of drugs, until her death in July 2011. She was [†]introduced to heroin and crack cocaine by her former husband, and is known to have [†]overdosed at least once on a mixture of heroin, crack, ecstasy, ketamine and alcohol. However, despite the media focus on her illicit drug use, it was her alcoholism that she struggled with most, and is probably what killed her in the end. It was the only drug found in her system when she died, alongside traces of Librium, which is commonly used to help alcoholics through withdrawal; her father claims that [†]she had seizures while attempting to stop drinking shortly before she died, and it's well known that these can be fatal.

Drugs – without the hot air, David Nutt

Psychological treatments

Psychological treatments try to help people understand how and why their addiction began, and use that understanding to avoid relapse or reduce harm. Probably the best known psychological treatment is the 12-step programme, which began with Alcoholics Anonymous but now has branches for everything from methamphetamine addiction to "emotional dependence". The programme helps people towards abstinence by taking them through a highly-structured process for rebuilding their lives, including making amends to those they've hurt through their addiction. Alcoholics Anonymous was begun by Christians, and although 12-step groups are not officially Christian organisations, they do use religious terminology, referring to a "higher power" which can help those who feel powerless over their compulsion to resist cravings. Whether or not anything supernatural is going on, this approach is clearly helpful to some people, (and more generally, being religious is protective against addiction).

There are also branches attached to many "anonymous" groups for the friends and families of addicts, and going through the process together can help everyone to re-establish contact and rebuild trust. The programme views addiction as a lifelong illness, but one which it is possible to resist through social support and willpower. The programme's focus on abstinence, however, can alienate those who find they cannot avoid relapse, sending them back into chaos if they fail to stay "clean".

A different psychological treatment is cognitive behavioural therapy (CBT). CBT identifies the internal, mental, social and environmental triggers that lead to drug taking, and develops coping strategies to avoid triggers leading to relapse. Some of the skills learned are practical – for example avoiding certain places and situations; others are internal – such as managing cravings by trying to remember the negative effects of the drug; and others are interpersonal – such as learning to say "no" convincingly to offers of drugs or alcohol. The addict learns to plan how to handle stressful situations and emergencies, and the possibility of "failure" is incorporated into the recovery plan. By preparing psychologically for the challenges the addict will inevitably face, it is hoped they will establish better coping mechanisms than by relying on willpower alone.

Other common psychological treatments include individual, couples or family therapy, where the environmental causes of the addiction can be discussed and dealt with. If the environment doesn't change, treatment is unlikely to work: for example, if someone is drinking to cope with a violent partner or family member, they are unlikely to stop while they remain in the abusive situation. Alternative sources of enjoyment are encouraged, such as taking up a sport or looking after a pet. Engaging in helping others with addiction is also a popular way of keeping off alcohol or drugs.

When people have multiple complex problems like this, practical support is an essential part of treatment. For most "problem drug users", their addiction is just one of a catalogue of difficulties in their lives, which they struggle with alongside a mixture of mental and physical health problems, extreme poverty and homelessness, social isolation and periods in and out of prison. Many will have had parents with similar problems, and will have had extremely deprived childhoods or been brought up in care. Many addiction treatment centres will link people up with services that can help with practical issues – women's shelters, or people who can provide specialist help with job seeking to facilitate leaving the sex trade. (One of the reasons opiates and crack cocaine are so widely used by prostitutes, and why many users become prostitutes, is that these drugs remove the disgust of sex with strangers. If an addict stops taking drugs but doesn't have the option of a different job, this may make life unbearable.)

In the chaos of many addicts' lives, psychological treatment may not be effective until their drug use has become more regular and stable. It is also extremely difficult to give someone therapy while they are either on drugs or in withdrawal, because they are too agitated and distressed. Keeping weekly appointments with a therapist may be all but impossible for somebody who has very little structure or schedule to their lives. Pharmacological substitutes, such as methadone or buprenorphine for heroin, have an important role to play in stabilising people to the point where psychological treatment can be effective; we explore these substitutes next.

Pharmacological substitutes

All behavioural addictions hijack our systems of motivation and reward, leading to repetitive behaviour even when it is clearly causing a great deal of harm. But drugs have an extra mechanism that drives people towards repeated use – the development of physical dependence and withdrawal. In the previous chapter we outlined Jim Orford's theory that drug addictions start with seeking pleasure but over time turn into a vicious cycle of trying to avoid withdrawal. Pharmacological substitutes are less harmful drugs that target the same receptors as the drug being abused, providing a mechanism for breaking this cycle, and making it easier for the patient to get off the drug of abuse when they are ready.

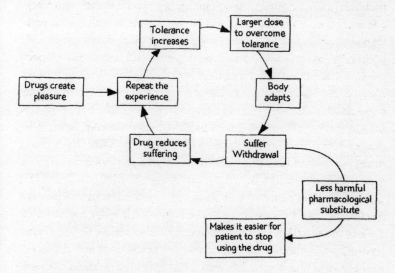

Figure 9.1: Pharmacological substitutes can help break the cycle of withdrawal.

There are two types of substitutes:

- *Full agonists.* A substitute agonist is a chemical that fits the receptors in the brain as precisely as the drug of abuse itself, but that is less harmful (either because it produces a lesser but longer-acting "high" or because it can be taken by a safer method). Nicotine gum and patches, and methadone, work in this way.
- *Partial agonists* fit the receptors in the brain well enough to avoid withdrawal, but without producing so much of a high. Whereas the full agonist nicotine gum produces the same high as a cigarette, the partial agonist varenicline (Champix) stops withdrawal and mimics a low level of smoking so the person feels as though they've smoked enough. This makes it an easier sort of substitute to stop using than a full agonist, which is inevitably going to be as addictive as the drug itself. Buprenorphine is a partial agonist for heroin, and we cover its use in detail later in this chapter.

Other pharmacological treatments

There are other sorts of drugs that can be used to treat addiction:

- *Antagonists.* These block the effects of the drug altogether, so that there is much less temptation to use it. For example, rimonabant blocks the cannabis receptors, making cannabis ineffective. Naltrexone stops heroin working, and can be used to prevent opiate addiction if users take it regularly; long-acting preparations including depot injections can make this easier. (For some people with opioid addiction, taking naltrexone can be made a condition of their continuing to work. For example, requiring addicted doctors and pharmacists to take naltrexone reduces the risk of their misappropriating supplies of drugs in their workplace.) A new kind of antagonist is the vaccine, which we'll discuss in chapter 16.
- *Pseudo-antagonists.* Whereas antagonists just block the positive effects of drugs, pseudo-antagonists actually produce negative effects. For example, Antabuse mimics the oriental flushing reaction to alcohol, by blocking the person's ability to break down the acetaldehyde that alcohol is converted into. When people drink

Drugs – without the hot air, David Nutt

after taking Antabuse they feel quite unwell and so get put off drinking any more. As we learn more about the biological factors which are protective against addiction, we will be able to develop more of these sorts of treatments.

- *Disease-modifying agents.* These are drugs that can stop aspects of addiction that lead to relapse. A good example is acamprosate (Campral) which reduces conditioned craving for alcohol. Some [†]opioid antagonists, including nalmefene and naltrexone, are now being used to reduce the effects of drinking so that bingeing is lessened. The possibility of developing [†]drugs to reduce stress-induced drug relapse is currently under investigation.

The development of the heroin-substitutes methadone and buprenorphine illustrates how substitutes can reduce the harm done by drug addiction. In the next sections we examine how heroin works in the body, how the substitutes operate, and why they can be effective as treatments.

What is heroin?

Heroin targets our endorphin receptors more effectively than almost any other drug, making it one of the most powerful painkillers we know of. Most of the world's supply is produced in Afghanistan and South East Asia; a small number of licensed companies produce medical-grade heroin, but the rest arrives on the streets as a brown solid which can be smoked or "cooked up" into a liquid using simple household items. This liquid is then put in a syringe and injected into veins, muscle or skin.

Heroin was first synthesised in 1874 and named heroin for its "heroic" subjective effects. It was marketed at first as a cough medicine and as a non-addictive alternative to morphine, but was soon found to be even more habit-forming. Its main effects are a sense of dreamy well-being, detachment and lack of concern about life's problems, and the absence of physical pain. It is used medicinally as a treatment for extreme pain and acute heart failure.

The drug itself causes little physical damage to the body, apart from chronic constipation. However, it causes severe damage indirectly:

- There is a high rate of overdosing among heroin users, because the combination of its low safety ratio and the fact that the street supply is of varying strengths, makes it hard for people to judge the correct dose.
- Heroin depresses breathing, and many heroin users take benzodiazepines or alcohol at the same time; both of which depress breathing further, and this can lead to death from low oxygen levels.
- Those who inject put themselves at risk of: HIV and hepatitis C from dirty needles; accidentally injecting lethal spores of bugs like anthrax and clostridium; and a range of other health issues such as skin infections and damaged veins.
- Pain sensations are suppressed, so that bad teeth, or being too hot or cold, can go unnoticed, which in turn can cause illnesses.
- Many addicts also suffer general ill health from heavy smoking, alcohol consumption and poor diet.

The social costs of these medical problems, disrupted family lives and crimes committed to feed addicts' habits are extremely high.

Why do people take heroin, and why can't they stop?

Many people start taking heroin to deal with physical or psychological pain – they may live in very deprived or unpleasant circumstances, or have experienced trauma such as child abuse or violence. Even when using heroin starts as pleasure seeking, the withdrawal syndrome is so severe that once the habit is formed it can be almost impossible to break the cycle. This is confounded by the fact that heroin passes into and out of the brain very quickly, with the result that habitual users are constantly either high or in withdrawal (Figure 9.2).

The withdrawal syndrome, while not life-threatening, is extremely unpleasant and distressing, because the body experiences the opposite effects of the drug. Where heroin creates profound relaxation, in withdrawal addicts get muscle cramps and tremor, producing a symptom known as "restless legs". (This is where the phrase "kicking the habit" comes from). Constipation is replaced by diarrhoea, low blood pressure

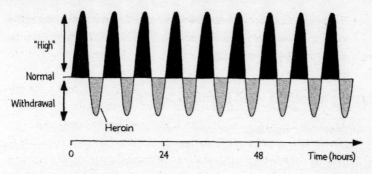

Figure 9.2: Heroin gets into and out of the brain very quickly, so the rapid high is swiftly followed by withdrawal.

with rapid pulse, drowsiness with insomnia, and a general sense of comfort and ease with fever and chills, gooseflesh, and irritability. This lasts for a week to ten days, and if an addict tries to detox without help when they still have access to heroin they will find it almost impossible to stop themselves taking it to end the nightmare of withdrawal.

If addicts don't know where their next hit is coming from – for example, if they don't have the money to buy it – they can become hugely distressed and possibly dangerous. As the beginning of withdrawal sets in, concern about the negative consequences of their actions is often overwhelmed by their desperate need to get the drug. The search for money can often lead to acquisitive crime – stealing from shops or from friends and family. This in turn leads to problems with the police, time in prison, and the erosion of the trust and support of those around them.

Physical detox is only the start of the struggle to stay off heroin. The psychological cravings can be exacerbated by an inability to feel pleasure from anything else, and this can last for months or years. If taking heroin was a response to trauma, having to relive the experience without the safety-net of the drug can be unbearable. Material deprivation and social isolation will undoubtedly have deteriorated since the habit began, and addicts may have few economic options outside crime and prostitution (especially if they have a criminal record for dealing, possession or stealing). Many heroin addicts say that the drug has long since ceased to give them any pleasure, and they are fully aware that it makes the chaos of their lives worse. But however miserable they may be on it, they are even more miserable without it.

Using heroin to treat heroin addicts

Until the 1960s, the "British model" of managing heroin addiction, used in the UK, was for addicts to be registered with doctors and prescribed heroin itself. This is still sometimes seen as the best approach, and has made a comeback in recent years in Switzerland. Users are given high-quality heroin which they inject with clean needles under medical supervision. There are signs that medicalising the whole experience has reduced some of the "rock star glamour" of the drug and helped reduce its appeal among the young.

The crucial advantage of prescribing heroin is that it's what the addict really *wants* to take, so they won't sell their supply to buy street drugs and will be highly motivated to continue treatment. Its main disadvantages are that users will continue to inject, and that its effects wear off so quickly they will continue to spend a lot of their time either high or waiting for their next fix. They no longer need to steal to fund their habit, are at much less risk of overdose, and won't get arrested for possession, but other chaotic aspects of their lifestyle are unlikely to improve.

Advantages and disadvantages of methadone treatment

In the 1950s, a new opioid called   methadone was developed, specifically as a substitute for heroin. This is a full agonist that stimulates the endorphin receptors as effectively as heroin does; however, it is broken down much more slowly in the body and is taken by mouth (a slower acting method than injection), so it creates a lesser high than heroin which lasts about 24 hours (Figure 9.3). During this time, methadone makes any heroin taken on top less effective (Figure 9.4), so the temptation to take heroin simultaneously is reduced.

Drugs – without the hot air, David Nutt

Methadone usually comes as green liquid that is swallowed under supervision at a clinic or pharmacy, although it is sometimes prescribed to be injected. The addict no longer has to commit crimes to fund their habit, can avoid withdrawal safely, and visiting the clinic every day gives some structure to their lives and access to other therapies. Having less of an up-and-down several times a day, and needing to spend less time drug seeking, makes it easier to rebuild relationships with family and to make practical arrangements for their lives. And anything that stops people injecting four times a day will reduce harm from infections; indeed, [†]methadone has been proved to reduce the spread of AIDS.

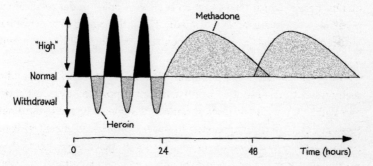

Figure 9.3: Methadone has a lower, slower, high than heroin. The methadone high lasts about 24 hours.

Methadone is far from perfect. Though safer than street-grade heroin, it still causes respiratory depression, and if users take heroin at the same time they are at serious risk of overdose. Some people manage to hold down jobs, but most long-term methadone users can't work as the drug leaves them somewhat "stoned", so they remain relatively deprived and socially isolated. The cheaper formulations are very sweet and can lead to loss of teeth, although there are sugar-free varieties. If methadone is left around the house, children sometimes drink it by mistake thinking it's syrup and can die. On weekdays these problems don't occur so much because the drug is taken at the clinic under supervision. However, at the weekend the addict is given two days' supply to take away, which is often injected contrary to what was intended, or sold to buy heroin. The

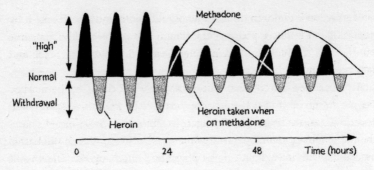

Figure 9.4: While methadone is in your system, it blocks on-top use of heroin, because any heroin you take will have a much lower effect than when on heroin alone.

final disadvantage of methadone is that its withdrawal syndrome is very painful and longer-lasting than heroin's.

Buprenorphine – a better solution?

Buprenorphine was developed as a painkiller in the 1990s, as a safer alternative to morphine. Its potential as a treatment for heroin addiction was soon recognised. It is sold under the trade name Subutex. Currently, about a quarter of all heroin addicts on pharmacological-substitute prescriptions are taking it, and it is the first-line treatment in France. As a partial agonist it is less pleasurable than heroin, but it also doesn't depress breathing so much, giving it a much higher safety ratio. It comes as a pill which is placed under the tongue and dissolves in saliva. (If swallowed, it gets absorbed by the liver and so doesn't work.) While it doesn't produce much of a high, it prevents withdrawal, and for an addict it is better than nothing. Also, like methadone, it blocks on-top heroin use.

Buprenorphine is an example of how good scientific research and feedback on addicts' behaviour in the real world can produce better treatments. Buprenorphine addresses several specific problems created by methadone: it lasts up to three days so there is no need to give take-away doses, so it is less likely to get diverted and sold on the street; it

Drugs – without the hot air, David Nutt

isn't sweet so if children do come across it they're unlikely to take it by accident, and if they do it won't kill them; and it doesn't knock people out the way methadone does, making it easier to hold down a job and take part in normal life.

A problem appeared when buprenorphine first came on the market: people dissolved it in water in order to inject it, often mixed with benzodiazepines, making it very dangerous. This also undermined one of the main aims of maintenance treatment, which is to reduce the harms associated with injecting. A clever pharmacological solution was to add the antagonist naloxone, which is inert if the pill is taken as directed under the tongue, but causes withdrawal if injected. The combination of buprenorphine and naloxone is sold under the name Suboxone.

Evaluating treatments

In the run-up to the UK 2010 general election, the Conservative party produced some provocative statements about long-term methadone treatment, arguing that taking it for just six weeks should be enough to get most heroin addicts stable enough to abstain. David Burrows, who was their spokesman on criminal justice at the time, was quoted saying [†]*"the public expects that addicts have to get off drugs but too many end up parked on methadone. They become dependent on it and end up not being able to contribute to their families or society."*

This attitude towards drug addiction derives from the views expressed in *Breakdown Britain*, a 2006 report by Iain Duncan Smith's think tank, the Centre for Social Justice. The report claimed that the addicts and counsellors it had spoken to thought that, for government-run services, abstinence was a better aim than harm reduction through controlled drinking or methadone treatment. It's unclear what their research methods were, as this viewpoint goes against [†]a substantial body of evidence which shows exactly the opposite. Although this hasn't been pursued as a policy since the coalition took power, it does mark a departure from the harm-reduction treatment model that the former Labour government were working with, which was one of the few areas of drug policy where they actually took on board evidence and expert advice.

One of the problems we face with addictions is that if abstinence is our only measure of success then none of the treatments we currently use are particularly successful. The very best long-term residential care – 3 to 4 months in a private addiction treatment clinic with access to psychological treatments and medical and pharmacological help – might lead to [†]40% of heroin addicts still being abstinent after year. Alcohol outpatient treatments have a far lower success rate – at best only [†]25% are still dry after twelve months.

Moreover, judging the success of a treatment on the outcome after 3 or 12 months isn't adequate. Addiction isn't a single transient event like a fractured bone or a chest infection, which can be "cured", in the sense that you will be no more prone to problems in the future than if it hadn't happened. Addiction is best thought of as a chronic recurring illness, like diabetes or asthma, where lifelong treatment is required. Once you've had an addiction you're always at greater risk of returning to it than those who have never been addicted, because you have an underlying vulnerability and your brain has changed as a result of repeated drug use. Longitudinal studies show lifetime relapse rates similar to asthma, diabetes or hypertension [†](Figure 9.5). As with these illnesses, relapse shouldn't be seen as a moral "failure". Instead, the most helpful attitude seems to be to re-evaluate the treatment model and maybe try something new.

There is no "one size fits all" model of treatment, because addiction has a great many different causes and all people are different. Some people may indeed be able to remain abstinent without any pharmacological substitutes. While this is the ideal, for others, attempting to stay "clean" makes the risk of relapse much higher, and pharmacological substitutes are necessary to reduce the chaos of their lives.

Fortunately, when we look beyond abstinence as the only measure of success, there are a great number of interventions that *can* reduce the harms caused by addiction. Since the costs of medical intervention are carried by the public, one good metric is economic – does this intervention save money overall? Given the enormous costs of problematic

Drugs – without the hot air, David Nutt

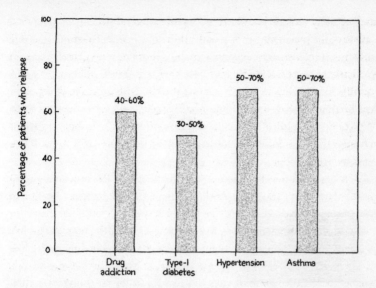

Figure 9.5: Relapse rates for drug-addicted patients are similar to those with other diseases.

heroin use (in treating HIV and hepatitis, taking children into care and policing acquisitive crime), methadone treatment is very cost-effective: [†]every pound of investment in methadone results in three pounds saved from these other sources. Buprenorphine is likely to be similarly cost-effective, and is probably better in the long term, though methadone may be better for stabilising people as it's more like heroin.

More generally, it's very important that this new generation of politicians appreciate the dynamics of addiction and don't return to the primitive, discredited moral model which is going out of fashion in the USA. Today's politicians have a different relationship to drugs than those in the past – many have acknowledged that they've tried cannabis and even Class A drugs like cocaine. Paradoxically, this may actually make them *less able* to understand the reality of addiction: since they tried these things once or several times, but then weighed up the pros and cons of continuing and had no trouble stopping, they think that other people should be able to do the same.

This view misses the point that these decisions are very different for addicts and non-addicts. A non-addict will probably find the threat of prison a pretty strong incentive not to steal to buy drugs – if they don't have enough money they'll go without. For a heroin or crack addict in withdrawal, prison is much less of a threat, and jail is actually a place where many peoples *start* their drug habits, rather than kicking them. In fact, it's hard to think of anything that would be an effective threat to someone with a serious addiction. Even if we brought in the death penalty for drug possession, as in Singapore, we would be unlikely to see all drug seeking cease – addicts often see friends and acquaintances injure themselves or die as a result of their habit, and that still doesn't stop them from using.

Just getting addicts into treatment in the first place is extremely challenging, and many simply won't come if the only outcome permitted is abstinence. It's pointless making policies assuming that people will behave how we want them to behave when we know they behave otherwise. We have to look at reality, decide what we want to achieve and what it is possible to achieve, and evaluate our policies honestly, in terms of our aims and any other perverse effects. One country which has done just that is Portugal.

The Portuguese experiment

In the 1980s and 90s, Portugal experienced a dramatic increase in the harms done by illegal drugs, in particular heroin. Although rates of drug use were lower overall than in other countries in Europe, almost all of those using heroin were seriously addicted, with the usual attendant problems of high rates of HIV and hepatitis, acquisitive crime and social disorder. By the end of the 20th century, [†]1% of the population were problematic drug users – 100,000 in a country of only 10 million – and it was recognised as the number one social problem. Pretty much everyone was personally affected by drug addiction, and there was a lot of interest in trying to find a new approach that would reduce harm.

In 1999, the Portuguese parliament approved a new National Strategy, which came into effect in 2001. Under this new strategy, drugs covered by the UN International Conventions remain illegal, but the penalties for personal use are no longer dealt with through the criminal justice system. Anyone caught with less than 10 days' average supply of a drug (5 g of cannabis, 1 g of heroin) has it confiscated by the police and they are given a ticket, requiring them to appear before a "dissuasion board" within 72 hours. The board is normally made up of two psychiatrists and a legal specialist, who ask about their drug use, categorise them as a recreational user or regular user or addict, warn them of the risks they are taking, and offer treatment if appropriate.

There are a range of potential sanctions, from a fine, to having social-security benefits cut or being forced to go to rehab. In practice though, about [†]85% of those sent to the board get a suspension with no sanctions, and most of the rest are given treatment. Supplying drugs is still penalised: if you're caught with more than 10 days' personal supply you still have to go to court and could face prison. A good comparison is with traffic offences: dangerous driving might land you in jail, but failing to wear a seat belt or cycling through a red light is more likely to result in a fine or having to go on a road-safety course.

Despite fears from some conservative politicians that decriminalisation would lead to a large increase in drug use, with Portugal becoming a site of "drug tourism", this has not happened and the policy has been highly successful at reducing harm, and has had few negative consequences:

- The [†]number of heroin addicts in treatment increased from 23,500 in 1998 to over 40,000 in 2010, partly due to the fact that they no longer have to fear criminal sanctions if they come forward.
- The number of new HIV cases among injecting drug users has reduced from [†]1,430 in 2000, to 352 in 2008.
- Halving the number of people injecting in the last month.
- Freeing up existing resources, which instead can be used to treat addiction and make larger seizures further up the supply chain.
- [†]Up to €400 million a year being taken out of the hands of criminals through decreased use.

Although there has been a slight increase in drug use among adults, there has been [†]a decrease among 15 to 19-year-olds, indicating lower levels of experimentation. This is very positive, because this was smaller than in neighbouring countries – Spain, for example – and drug behaviour in teenage years has a strong relationship with drug use later in life. Nor has Portugal become a destination for foreign drug users; [†]95% of those caught since the strategy was introduced have been Portuguese.

The most significant change, however, has been in the social attitude towards drug addiction. It is now seen primarily as a medical and social problem rather than a moral or criminal one. And far from the Portuguese state being "soft on drugs", they are intervening more than ever, taking steps to deter people from progressing from recreational use to addiction, and heavily encouraging people into treatment. There is also a recognition that a response which might work well for one person would be less effective for another, and that addicts respond to different sorts of incentives than non-addicts. Fines are specifically not recommended as a punishment for addicts, for example, lest they commit crimes to get the money to pay the fine.

Preventing addiction

Could addiction be prevented? There are certainly external factors that affect its prevalence, and there is a very close relationship between addiction and the price and availability of drugs: the cheaper and more available something is, the more addiction there will be. This applies to both legal and illegal drugs, and to behaviours such as gambling – in common with many other countries we've seen a substantial rise in gambling addictions in the UK since gambling laws were relaxed. Even addicts are price sensitive (though less so than non-addicts). Increasing the cost of cigarettes has caused many smokers to cut down, and although they remain addicted, smoking 10 a day is far less harmful than smoking 20. Before addiction sets in, price is even more influential at stopping people from taking drugs in the first place or going on to use them extensively. Obviously government regulation can't have any direct effect

Drugs – without the hot air, David Nutt

on the street price of illegal drugs, but taxing legal addictive substances is effective in reducing use and addiction.

Addiction is far more likely to occur when adverse initial effects are overcome. Ethanol is extremely unpleasant – the closest thing to it most of us drink is vodka, and few people drink that neat. When we want to make laboratory rats become alcoholics we give them a sweet solution (which they love) containing a small amount of alcohol, and gradually increase the alcohol concentration until they are dependent on the drug. This is essentially the process that alcopops replicate, and banning or controlling their sale may help to stop young people from developing drink problems.

Conclusion

This chapter opened with three contrasting stories about addiction: Tony Adams, who has succeeded in abstaining from alcohol for over a decade; Amy Winehouse, who's been killed by her alcohol use; and Pete Doherty, who seems unable to find a treatment for his addictions to heroin and crack and continues taking them even though he keeps harming himself and others. But Adams, even though he's a "success story", is still an alcoholic, although it's been many years since his last drink. His experience in Alcoholics Anonymous will have taught him that "once an addict, always an addict".

The Conservative party's *Breakdown Britain* report criticised Labour's policy on the treatment of addiction, saying that *"it has pushed treatment in the wrong direction, preferring maintenance (substitute prescription) to recovery."* This statement in itself betrays a lack of understanding of the mechanisms of addiction – there's no such thing as "recovery" from addiction in the way that you can "recover" from a broken arm. Abstinence itself could be described as a form of maintenance – someone who has been an addict is always at risk of relapse, and abstinence will require conscious maintenance. In any lifelong illness, different treatments may be effective at different times, and someone who finds themselves able to abstain for many years may find that stress or bereavement causes a relapse which is then best treated with a pharmacological substitute, at least for a period.

Even though, with our current medical knowledge, addiction can't be cured, there are still ways to reduce the harm that it causes, and there are treatments that can reduce the distress of the illness and make relapse less likely. To start, we must fully adopt the medical model of addiction, and discard the long-discredited moralistic one that blames the addict for their condition. When somebody develops diabetes, they may have made getting the disease more likely through their diet, but this doesn't mean that we would deny them insulin. Quite apart from the fact that many of the factors that put them at risk (such as their genes) were out of their control, there's also a humane recognition that even a self-induced illness should receive treatment.

It is questionable whether the medical model of addiction can ever really become accepted as long as possession of drugs for personal use carries criminal sanctions. Given the involuntary nature of drug-taking for many addicts, and the heavy penalties they suffer already, it's inhumane to put them through the criminal justice system for doing something over which they have very little control. The experience of Portugal shows that when policies are consistently based on the belief that a drug addict is a sick person, rather than a criminal or delinquent, huge improvements can be made in their lives, and to society as a whole. Rather than dismantling methadone treatment programs, which are a vital lifeline for some extremely vulnerable and disadvantaged people, perhaps our politicians should look across at the Portuguese example?

Notes

Page

155 Tony Adams• *Addicted*, Tony Adams & Ian Ridley, HarperCollinsWillow, 1998

156 a very public battle with heroin and crack addiction for over a decade.• *Pete Doherty jailed for six months*, Caroline Davies, URL-74, May 20th 2011

156 introduced to heroin and crack cocaine by her former husband• *Divorce Drama for Amy Winehouse*, Simon Perry, URL-75, December 1st 2008

Drugs – without the hot air, David Nutt

156 overdosed at least once• *Amy Winehouse bailed over drugs video*, Anita Singh, URL-76, May 8th 2008

156 she had seizures while attempting to stop drinking shortly before she died• *Amy Winehouse died after detox seizures, dad says*, Maria Puente, URL-77, September 10th 2011

161 opioid antagonists, including nalmefene and naltrexone, are now being used to reduce the effects of drinking• *Evidence-based guidelines for the pharmacological management of substance misuse, addiction and comorbidity: recommendations from the British Association for Psychopharmacology*, A R Lingford-Hughes, S Welch, D J Nutt, Journal of Psychopharmacology (18) 3, 2004

161 drugs to reduce stress-induced drug relapse• *Neurobiological mechanisms for opponent motivational processes in addiction*, George F Koob and Michel L Moal, in *The Neurobiology of Addiction*, Oxford University Press, 2010

165 methadone has been proved to reduce the spread of AIDS• *Substitution maintenance therapy in the management of opioid dependence and HIV/AIDS prevention*, WHO/UNODC/ UNAIDS, URL-78, 2004.

167 *"the public expects that addicts have to get off drugs but too many end up parked on methadone.•* *Will Conservative plans to overhaul heroin addiction treatment work?*, Denis Campbell, URL-79, April 20th 2010

167 a substantial body of evidence which shows exactly the opposite• *An overview of systematic reviews of the effectiveness of opiate maintenance therapies: available evidence to inform clinical practice and research*, Laura Amato et al, Journal of Substance Abuse 28 (4), 2005

168 40% of heroin addicts still being abstinent after year• *Factors associated with abstinence, lapse or relapse to heroin use after residential treatment: protective effect of coping responses*, Michael Gossop et al, Addiction (97), September 2002

168 25% are still dry after twelve months.• *How effective is alcoholism treatment in the United States?*, William Miller, Scott Walters and Melanie Bennett, Journal Studies of Alcohol (62), 2001. This paper noted that although only 1 in 4 remained continuously abstinent in the year following treatment, most of the remainder did drink less intensively, deriving some benefit from the treatment even if they weren't completely abstinent.

168 (Figure 9.5).• *Drugs, Brains, and Behavior: The Science of Addiction*, URL-169, NIDA, August 2010, which quotes source as JAMA 284:1689–1695, 2000

169 every pound of investment in methadone results in three pounds saved from these other sources• *Crutch or cure? The realities of methadone treatment*, David Nutt, URL-80, June 9th 2010

170 1% of the population were problematic drug users● Dr Joao Goulao, in a presentation first delivered at ISCD summit, November 2010

171 85% of those sent to the board get a suspension with no sanctions● *Drug Decriminalization in Portugal: lessons for creating fair and successful drug policies,* Glenn Greenwald, Cato Institute, URL-81, 2009

171 number of heroin addicts in treatment increased from 23,500 in 1998 to over 40,000 in 2010● *What Britain could learn from Portugal's drugs policy,* Peter Beaumont, URL-82, September 5th 2010

171 1,430 in 2000, to 352 in 2008● *Drug Policy in Portugal: the benefits of decriminalising drug use,* Artur Domaslawski, URL-83, June 2011

171 Up to €400 million a year being taken out of the hands of criminals● *What Britain could learn from Portugal's drugs policy,* Peter Beaumont, URL-82, September 5th 2010

172 a decrease among 15 to 19-year-olds● *Drug Decriminalization in Portugal: lessons for creating fair and successful drug policies,* Glenn Greenwald, Cato Institute, URL-81, 2009

172 95% of those caught since the strategy was introduced have been Portuguese● As above.

10 Cocaine – from chewing to crack (or, eats shoots and leaves)

This chapter is about the different forms in which drugs can be taken, and how that affects the harm they do, using cocaine as an example. The ways in which a drug can be taken depend on various properties: whether it's available as a solid, liquid or gas; whether it's soluble; and what its melting point is. The different methods used to deliver drugs to the brain are called *routes of use*, and the health impacts of a drug can vary enormously depending on how it's consumed.

Routes of use and main associated harms

Over the centuries, many different ways of taking drugs have been developed. In the first instance plants were chewed or eaten, or in the case of alcohol, fermented into a liquid and drunk. Smoking developed with tobacco and then cannabis – when the practice came to Europe it was so alien that for a long time is was still referred to as "drinking". Once purification of the chemical components of drugs had been achieved, the pure forms were taken either as pills or tinctures, or in the case of gases inhaled; and eventually, after the invention of the hypodermic syringe, injected. The seven most common routes of use and the principal sorts of harm they do are:

1. *Chewing* is the slowest route into the brain, with levels of the drug generally peaking 1–2 hours after chewing begins. Regular chewers of drugs such as khat, coca leaves and nicotine gum, can develop tooth, gum and jaw problems.
2. *Drinking and eating*. The drug generally takes effect after about 30 minutes. Sometimes this delay means that users find it hard to

judge when they've had enough, increasing the risk of overdose. This is why people taking strong alcoholic drinks can get extremely drunk so easily.

3. *Rubbing* onto membranes such as gums, eyelids and genitals, is effective in 15–30 minutes. This can cause infections and necrosis. When stimulants are frequently rubbed into gums, the teeth can start to fall out as their blood supply is cut off.

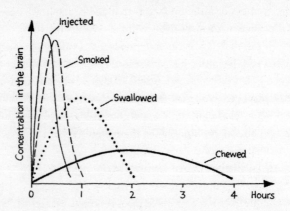

Figure 10.1: How the route of use affects the speed and intensity of a drug's effect.

4. *Snorting* hits the brain in 3 to 5 minutes. Compulsive snorters of drugs like cocaine can seriously damage their noses, getting nasal ulcers or perforating their septums.

5. *Shooting* or injecting can be done into veins (which hits the brain in 10–20 seconds) or into muscle (3–5 minutes). It is associated with a range of related harms, such as skin and other bacterial infections, viruses such as hepatitis and HIV, and also thrombosis and the risk of sudden death.

6. *Smoking* is another very quick route, hitting the brain in 10–20 seconds. Tobacco smoke is carcinogenic and smoking of all kinds can cause respiratory problems such as asthma and emphysema.

7. *Inhaling* is the route of use for gases such as butane and liquid solvents, which reach the brain within seconds, and the heart even

Drugs – without the hot air, David Nutt

faster than that. Inhalants can cause sudden heart and breathing failure and death.

Figure 10.1 shows schematically the relative speeds of the most common routes of use.

Why are drugs used in different forms?

There are a number of different factors that determine how successful or harmful a particular form of drug will be. Within the industries, both legal and illegal, there are economic pressures to deliver the biggest hit of a drug per unit weight. This is particularly so for illegal drugs, which must be smuggled large distances around the world, but the drinks industry has also been gradually increasing the alcohol content of beers, ciders and wine. Ensuring that people consume more of the drug with every sip will almost certainly make these alcoholic drinks more addictive, guaranteeing a very reliable market.

Drugs are usually consumed within a social context, and some forms are seen as more sociable because they are easier to share. Cannabis is an obvious example because it is passed from person to person when it is being smoked; however it's much harder to share cannabis this way when it is being eaten. (Similarly, tobacco smokers are unlikely to ask if they could share a nicotine patch, but will often ask each other for cigarettes.) On the other hand, it's much harder to be discreet when smoking, and in many contexts drugs are unacceptable even if they're legal. A cannabis cookie is more discreet than a spliff, and spirits are easier to drink surreptitiously than beer – the hip-flask for spirits being popular for precisely this reason.

Kinetics and dynamics of addiction

There are the two measures that determine how addictive a drug is:

- *Kinetics* involves the route of use, which largely determines the *speed of onset*, ie how quickly a drug takes effect, and the *speed of offset*, ie how quickly it wears off. Both faster onset and faster offset tend to increase the addictiveness of a drug. Figure 10.2 shows the relative speed of entry into the brain of various drugs in different forms.

- *Dynamics* is a measure of the *efficacy* of the drug in the brain – how efficient it is at binding with the receptors or enzymes it targets. The greater the efficacy, the greater the addictive potential.

(In other words, the kinetics specifies how the drug moves in and out of the brain, while the dynamics is what it does when it gets there.)

Kinetics often has an effect on a drug's legal Class. When amphetamine sulphate is sold as a powder, which has a high melting point and can't be smoked, it's a Class B drug, whereas methamphetamine, which has a lower melting point and *can* be smoked, is in Class A. Similarly, when amphetamine sulphate is sold in ampoules as a liquid which can be injected, it's also placed in Class A. This is a good example of how the classification system of the Misuse of Drugs Act *can* give people accurate information about relative harm. Injecting any drug always carries more risks than snorting it or taking it orally (because of the risk of contracting blood-borne viruses and infections when injecting). It makes sense for methamphetamine and liquid amphetamine to be in a higher Class than amphetamine powder, because the former *are* more harmful.

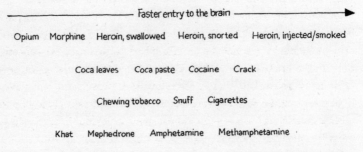

Figure 10.2: Faster entry to the brain gives quicker effects and makes a drug more addictive.

Drugs – without the hot air, David Nutt

From chewing to crack: the history of cocaine

Cocaine illustrates how the kinetics of a drug can determine the harm that it does, since it can now be consumed by almost every route of use, with varying kinetics. The journey from coca leaf (from which cocaine was originally derived) to crack (which is a particularly dangerous form of cocaine) shows how a non-addictive substance can be modified to make one of the most addictive drugs ever known, largely by changing how it reaches the brain. It also shows how international drug policies, even when brought in with the best intentions, can have perverse effects, leading to environmental destruction, political collapse, huge profits for criminal gangs and the arrival of even more harmful substances on our streets. Let's now look at the progress of cocaine in detail.

Coca in the Andes

Cocaine is [†]the psychoactive component of the coca plant, in which it acts as a natural insecticide. Coca is native to the foothills of the Andes of Peru and Bolivia, where it has been used by indigenous people for thousands of years, although most of the world's supply is now grown in Colombia. Coca chewing is an important part of indigenous culture, with a wide variety of uses as a medicine, in religious rituals and in social life. Coca leaves are presented in marriage ceremonies, chewed at feasts, help people work for long periods at high altitudes, and also contain vitamins and minerals which are an important part of local diets.

Dried coca leaves are mixed with lime to form a "quid" which is placed between the cheek and gum, and sucked. The lime helps extract the cocaine from the leaves, but the process is very slow, and peak concentrations in the brain are only reached after about two hours. Because the effect happens so slowly, users rarely experience psychological cravings if they stop, although if they rely on it to deal with physical hardship they will, of course, feel worse if they don't chew it any more. Coca chewers are not addicted to cocaine.

When the Spanish conquistadors encountered coca in the 1500s, it fascinated and quite alarmed them. The Catholic Church disapproved of its use in Shamanic rituals, and [†]in 1569 they declared that it had satanic powers and that all plantings should be destroyed. The colonists soon discovered, however, that the indigenous people were much less productive when they didn't have coca's stimulating effects, particularly in the silver and gold mines where they often refused to work without their coca rations. In the end, the Spanish accepted the importance of the practice, and began profiting from the trade by levying a 10% tax on coca sales.

Cocaine comes to Europe

Numerous attempts were made to transport coca back to Europe, but the leaves had usually lost their potency by the time they'd crossed the Atlantic. It wasn't until two new and far stronger forms appeared in the mid-1800s that it became widely used by Europeans. The first was pure cocaine hydrochloride, which was extracted and isolated by Friedriche Gaedecke in 1855. The second appeared in 1863, when French chemist Angelo Mariani hit upon the idea of fortifying alcohol with coca leaves to produce [†]"Vin Mariani". This was about 10% alcohol and 8.5% cocaine; it was marketed as a tonic capable of preventing illnesses such as stomach and lung troubles, malaria and influenza, "giving life and vigour ... invaluable for all bodily and mental overexertions". It became hugely popular, with fans as eminent as Queen Victoria, and Pope Leo XIII who appeared in an advertisement for the drink (Figure 10.3) and even awarded it a Vatican gold medal.

Meanwhile, the medical establishment was trying to work out whether this "wonder drug" had real therapeutic uses. In 1884, Freud began experimenting with it as a cure for depression and morphine addiction, realising only belatedly that it was almost as addictive as morphine. It was his colleague Karl Koller who in the same year recognised its first genuine medical application as a local anaesthetic for eye and nose surgery, since it both dulls pain and constricts blood vessels, minimising blood loss. Although a vast improvement on previous sorts of anaesthetics, this could also be dangerous, as wads of cocaine which had been put up the nose were sometimes swallowed by mistake, resulting in heart attacks.

Drugs – without the hot air, David Nutt

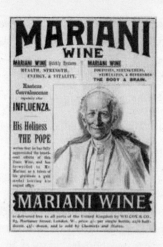

Figure 10.3: Pope Leo XIII endorsed Mariani Wine.

Self-experimentation was a common form of scientific research at the time, and some doctors and scientists snorted or injected large amounts, while others made it into a paste and applied to almost every part of the body they could think of. Many developed chronic cocaine addictions as they investigated its physical and psychological properties.

Cocaine was everywhere. Injecting cocaine intravenously (famously practised by Sherlock Holmes) was relatively common, and considered pretty unremarkable. Another widely-available form of cocaine, which became hugely popular in the USA, was in a fizzy soft drink. In 1886, perhaps inspired by Mariani, a chemist from Atlanta called John Pemberton created his own alcohol and coca leaf concoction called Pemberton's †French Wine Coca. When Atlanta brought in prohibition later that year, he removed the alcohol and began selling his unique combination of cocaine, kola nut (which provided a dose of caffeine), corn syrup and soda water, which became a huge temperance hit under the name Coca-Cola. Soda fountains sprang up all over the city and became very popular.

Pemberton sold the company to a devout teetotaler who started using "decocainised" leaves to flavour the drink as soon as it became clear that the drug was addictive. In fact, the biggest battle the Coca-Cola company faced was over its caffeine content, involving a very high-profile [†]court case against the American government to prove that caffeine was not deleterious to health.

Understanding cocaine

By the early 1900s, the properties of cocaine, including its harms, were starting to be better understood. In overdose, it constricts the blood vessels in the heart, which can cause heart attacks, seizures, pulmonary oedema (fluid in the lungs) or can rupture the aorta. Sometimes heavy use results in a condition called myocardial fibrosis, where normal heart muscle is replaced with fibrous tissue so the heart can't pump blood properly, and cocaine can also increase thromboxane production, causing blood clots. Regular use can lead to psychosis, with paranoia, delusions, and a symptom called formication (the phantom sensation of ants or insects crawling across the skin). Snorting large amounts can lead to ulcers in the nose or a perforated septum due to loss of blood supply because the drug constricts the blood vessels. Regularly injecting into sensitive areas like genitals can lead to necrosis, where the skin dies, which in severe cases can only be treated with amputation. [†]Using cocaine while pregnant can cause problems for the foetus, and carries an eight times higher risk of Sudden Infant Death Syndrome.

None of these health problems are seen to a significant degree among coca chewers, nor does coca lead to compulsive use and addiction. Cocaine blocks dopamine reuptake in the brain, resulting in an increase in dopamine, but chewing allows these effects to build up to a much lesser extent, and to reduce gradually, so the brain has time to adapt. Cocaine hydrochloride, which can be snorted, injected or pasted on skin, can reach the brain much more quickly, creating a faster rush, bigger high, and bigger crash as the brain tries to readjust. As discussed in chapter 8, the brain's reaction to big increases in dopamine is often to reduce the number of functioning dopamine receptors, leading to a reduced sense of reward from other activities and greater dependence on the drug.

Cocaine wine (Vin Mariani) is also more potent and addictive than coca, as it combines cocaine and alcohol, which together react to form cocaethylene. This compound is even more harmful than either alcohol or cocaine on their own, so people drinking cocaine wine are essentially consuming three powerfully addictive drugs at once – no wonder it was so popular!

Crack in the cities

The backlash against cocaine led to ever stricter controls during the first half of the 20th century, until its outright prohibition and a concerted international effort to reduce production as part of the War on Drugs. This was partially successful at first, but the reduction in supply wasn't accompanied by a decrease in demand in the West, causing the price of cocaine to sky-rocket. The increase in international border controls, and rise in costs as large volumes of the drug were seized, led to producers trying to develop cheaper forms of cocaine that would be easier to transport. The result was [†]crack, which appeared in the USA in 1984.

Crack is the *freebase* form of cocaine, ie the base organic substance (rather than the salt that is formed when the organic base reacts with hydrochloric acid), although it usually isn't entirely "pure", [†]because of how it is produced. Hydrochlorides are more stable compounds so they tend to be the form street drugs take, but they usually can't be smoked because they vaporise at such high temperatures that they burn instead, and become useless. Crack vaporises at 90°; cocaine hydrochloride vaporises at 190°, and in air will burn and lose its efficacy before it can reach this temperature.

Along with the lung problems that always accompany regular smoking, crack users are more likely to experience psychosis, aggression and heart failure, and are much more likely to escalate into habitual use and addiction. On pretty much every measure of harm, our expert panel rated crack as more harmful than cocaine, but particularly on crime, and loss of tangibles and relationships. This reflects the fact that crack has become popular amongst a similar poor, urban demographic as those who take up heroin, and in fact the term "problem drug user" generally now refers to heroin and crack addicts. Whereas non-crack cocaine tends to be used by people in employment who fund their drug use out of wages,

	Crack cocaine	Cocaine
Route of use	smoking	injecting/snorting
Speed of onset	10 seconds	15–30 seconds (injecting) 1–3 minutes (snorting)
Speed of offset	15 minutes	15–20 mins (injecting) 30 minutes (snorting)
Drug efficacy	high	high

Table 10.1: The kinetics of crack and cocaine.

crack is often funded through crime, leading to the same spiral of loss of trust with family and friends, marginalisation, and periods in and out of prison as we see with heroin. Although not as widespread as opiates, at least in the UK, crack has torn apart communities and destroyed many people's lives. (The TV series *The Wire* gives a realistic and visual account of the damage that crack causes.)

Why is crack twice as addictive as cocaine?

As we said, the addictiveness of a drug is determined by both kinetics (how a drug gets to the brain) *and* what it does when it gets there. When our expert panel was considering the addictiveness of the 20 drugs, crack was rated at 100, along with heroin, while cocaine powder when snorted was given a score of 50. This shows how important kinetics is: since cocaine powder and crack have identical dynamic effects, the difference in addictiveness is almost entirely due to kinetics: crack can be smoked.

Smoking crack cocaine results in a faster high and swifter come down than snorting or injecting cocaine powder (Figure 10.1 and Table 10.1), making it significantly more likely to cause dependence. Once in the brain, the two forms of the drug have identical effects.

Cocaine powder is expensive compared with other "party drugs" such as ecstasy and amphetamines, but it has a less obvious form of intoxication, making it more socially acceptable outside of clubs. It encourages self-interested, aggressive and risk-taking behaviour, and is popular among people employed in areas such as the media and high finance,

Drugs – without the hot air, David Nutt

where these personality traits are often associated with success (or with financial disasters, in more recent years!). In these highly competitive environments, there's often a lack of trust, and groups may become socially dependent on the drug as a social lubricant, usually alongside heavy drinking. Although the price has dropped in recent years, its expense still makes it a bit of a status symbol, and large doses are sometimes taken as an explicit sign of wealth and prestige. Because cocaine both induces anti-social behaviour and makes users less concerned for the welfare of others, what begins as an experience sought after for its pleasurable effects can also become the means of escaping the social consequences of actions while intoxicated. The cocaine user can get caught in a cycle of egotistical and self-interested behaviour when "high", that then drives them back to the drug in order to minimise feelings of regret or remorse.

Crack cocaine, in contrast, is relatively cheap, and it's associated with poverty and areas of social deprivation. The aggression and risk-taking of cocaine is amplified with crack; it has become an important social tool in some gang cultures, helping young men to psych themselves up before acts of violence and dissociate themselves from feelings of regret. The sense of invincibility created by the drug can be psychologically useful in dangerous and hostile social environments, fuelling addiction.

Conclusion

What do the story of cocaine, and drug kinetics in general, tell us about reducing the harm done by drugs? Virtually all the harms caused by cocaine don't occur when it is released very slowly into the brain by chewing: coca leaf doesn't cause heart problems or addiction, and avoids the nose and lung problems caused by snorting or smoking. So it's not necessarily a drug *itself* that is the source of harm, but the route of use and the drug's social context. The safety of coca chewing and its place in Bolivian culture are why the President of Bolivia recently withdrew his country's support for the UN convention on cocaine, to allow coca chewing to become legal again in Bolivia.

This poses some interesting questions. Should we encourage certain sorts of drug-taking in order to discourage more harmful behaviour? Although smoking carries its own dangers, it's definitely less harmful than injecting – should intravenous heroin users be persuaded to change to smoking instead? Or perhaps there are ways to reverse the process where drugs become available in more potent and more addictive forms over time. It's unlikely that coca chewing would become popular in the UK, but maybe a weak sort of cocaine drink or cocaine tea could be developed, as a less harmful alternative to cocaine powder or crack?

The story of cocaine also illustrates that we need to find an approach to drugs which neither involves making them freely available in the shops, nor prohibiting them altogether and driving the trade into the black market. When cocaine was legally available as a salt, and was being widely consumed in Mariani wine, there was a significant increase in harm and addiction, which we certainly don't want repeated. But since international prohibition, we've seen not only environmental destruction and huge profits handed to criminal gangs and corrupt governments, but also the invention of crack, an even more addictive and deadly form of the drug, as a direct result of the economic pressures of forcing the trade underground. Addiction is one of the greatest hazards of drug use, and harm reduction measures must always have reducing addiction as a principal aim.

The international damage done by cocaine

When our expert panel ranked the 20 drugs for "international damage", it was quickly decided [†]to give cocaine and crack the maximum score of 100. Although heroin wasn't far behind, cocaine was judged as having caused more harm overall – to the people in producer countries such as Bolivia and Colombia, and in intermediary countries involved in the trade like Mexico and Guinea-Bissau.

The problems begin at the plantations. The majority of coca leaf is produced by small-scale farmers with few other options for earning a living. Growing coca is preferable to other crops because it has a higher market value, and because it plays an important part in social life. It

Drugs – without the hot air, David Nutt

can also grow on difficult terrain, and when it's cultivated using traditional and sustainable farming techniques, it can improve soil quality by binding it together with its roots. Unfortunately, the policy of destroying coca plantations in order to reduce the global cocaine supply means that farmers have to focus on getting the maximum yield in the short term, using techniques which degrade the soil, and they are forced to clear more rainforest when their crops are burnt or sprayed with herbicide chemicals. It's been estimated that [†]every gram of cocaine snorted in the UK will have been responsible for 4 square metres of rainforest being destroyed in Colombia or the Amazon, creating local environmental problems and contributing to climate change by reducing one of the world's biggest carbon sinks.

The farmers sell the coca to the organisations that manufacture cocaine; these may be criminal cartels, revolutionary forces, corrupt state employees or covert government-approved groups, who maintain the official line that they're clamping down on production while actually supporting it. In Colombia, control of cocaine production has become a major factor in the ongoing violence between government and paramilitary forces and the Revolutionary Armed Forces of Colombia (FARC), both of which draw large amounts of revenue from the trade. Farmers are often caught in the middle, having to make difficult decisions about who to sell their crop to, which adds to the insecurity they already experience because of the large price fluctuations.

The manufacturing process to turn coca into cocaine causes even more problems than the plantations. Illicit factories, laboratories and maceration pits, which are often hidden in the rainforest, dump toxic chemicals such as kerosene, ether and sulphuric acid, contaminating soil and water supplies. Obviously, these can't be regulated by any kind of environmental legislation because they operate outside the law. However, the government organisations that pursue the cocaine manufacturers also have little regard for the local environment, and cause just as much pollution when they launch operations against these factories, destroying buildings and machinery but leaving the hazardous chemicals on site.

Aside from environmental destruction in producer countries, the trade also causes political and social problems in the transit countries the drug passes through before it arrives in the places that consume it. The majority of the world's cocaine is consumed in North America and Europe, and is channelled to them via Mexico and West Africa respectively. Mexico has seen the development of extremely powerful cartels, and there is evidence that they are now controlling large-scale production in Colombia as well, not just acting as middlemen. A government-led crackdown on these cartels, which began in 2006, seems to have exacerbated the violence, with nearly [†]35,000 deaths attributed to the drugs war since then, 15,000 of them in 2010 alone. Most of these have taken place in cities along the northern border between Mexico and the USA, and this border has become one of the most dangerous places in the world. Since the mid-2000s, much of the cocaine being consumed in Europe has started to be[†] channelled through unstable states in West Africa such as Guinea Bissau, undermining the development of democratic institutions or attempts by civil society organisations to tackle corruption within governments and the police.

In this huge, unregulated trade, millions of other people are harmed: the children used as sentries to watch out for law enforcement agencies, the people coerced into acting as drug mules, the bystanders killed during cartel turf wars, the citizens who lose out on health and education because their governments are corrupted by drug money or are spending billions on fighting drug production. None of these policies have reduced demand for the drug, which has an estimated 17 million users worldwide. Minimising the harms done by cocaine needs to take into account the international aspects of the trade, and work towards solutions that reduce the insecurity and violence which accompanies it. As long as demand for the drug exists, so will cocaine production. Finding a way of regulating it to avoid the terrible level of collateral damage will probably be impossible as long as prohibition is the only policy option available.

Drugs – without the hot air, David Nutt

Notes

Page

181 the psychoactive component of the coca plant• *20 (mis)conceptions on coca and cocaine*, Roberto Laserna, Plural Publishers, 1997

182 in 1569 they declared that it had satanic powers• *20 (Mis)conceptions on coca and cocaine*, Roberto Laserna, Plural Publishers, 1997

182 "Vin Mariani"• *High Society*, Mike Jay, Thames & Hudson, 2010

183 French Wine Coca• *QI: quite interesting facts about wine*, John Mitchinson and Molly Oldfield, URL-84, December 17th 2009

184 court case against the American government• *United States v. Forty Barrels and Twenty Kegs of Coca-Cola*, 241 US 265, 1916

184 Using cocaine while pregnant can cause problems for the foetus, and carries an eight times higher risk of Sudden Infant Death Syndrome• *Illegal drugs: a complete guide to their history, chemistry, use and abuse*, Paul M Ghalinger, Plume, 2003

185 crack, which appeared in the USA in 1984• *DEA History Book*, 1876–1990 (drug usage & enforcement), US Department of Justice, 1991

185 because of how it is produced.• Freebase can be made from cocaine powder (which is cocaine hydrochloride) using chemical extraction (eg with ether) in which case it is pure, or from cocaine extract that is not purified to powder, and then left in an impure state with some of the processing chemicals (alkali salts) still present in the mixture. Using ether is more difficult and dangerous for manufacturers, so they usually opt for the second process. The Wikipedia article *Crack cocaine* (URL-85) has more detail on the chemistry.

188 to give cocaine and crack the maximum score of 100.• *20 (mis)conceptions on coca and cocaine*, Roberto Laserna, Plural Publishers, 1997

189 every gram of cocaine snorted in the UK will have been responsible for 4 square metres of rainforest being destroyed in Colombia or the Amazon• *Cocaine users are destroying the rainforest – at 4 square metres a gram*, Sandra Leville, URL-86, November 19th 2008

190 35,000 deaths attributed to the drugs war since then• *Mexico updates four years of drug war deaths to 34,612*, BBC News, URL-87, January 13, 2011. The estimate is now 40,000.

190 channelled through unstable states in West Africa such as Guinea Bissau• *War on Drugs: Report of the Global Commission on Drugs Policy*, URL, June 2011

11 Why was smoking banned in public places?

The 2007 ban on smoking in public places in the UK

On July 1st 2007, England became the last nation in the United Kingdom to ban smoking in public places. With some minor exceptions, any substantially-enclosed place would now have to display "no smoking" signs and take steps to stop people from lighting up. [†]Individuals who broke the ban would face a £50 fine, while owners could be charged £2,500 for failing to prevent smoking on their premises. Despite the media depicting the ban as "controversial", [†]three quarters of adults supported the legislation before it was brought in, and support has remained high ever since.

Many places were already no-smoking by 2007, but without a blanket ban there would always be exceptions, and the dangers of second-hand smoke were thought to be sufficiently high to justify the inconvenience to smokers. There was particular concern about effects on the health of people working in pubs and bars, and a desire to dissociate smoking and drinking as part of a general effort to make cigarettes seem less normal. It was also hoped that cleaner environments would help current smokers to quit, and perhaps prevent some people from starting.

Keeping places smoke free is just one of the public-health measures introduced in the last 50 years to reduce smoking. Others have included restrictions on tobacco advertising, warnings on cigarette packets, raising the age of sale to 18, and increasing the price through taxes. In 2011, the British government announced plans to ban the display of cigarettes in shops, and announced that they were considering a ban on any kind of branding, requiring plain generic packaging instead. All these measures have been fiercely resisted by the tobacco industry, but they have undoubtedly had a positive effect on the health of the nation: the proportion of British adults who smoke has dropped from about [†]40% in 1978 to about 20% today, saving thousands of lives. Many of the regulations I've suggested for reducing the harms of alcohol are inspired by the successes of the tobacco control movement. The story of tobacco is a paradigm case of what happens when drug companies are allowed to create markets of millions of addicts, and what governments can do to rein in those markets without making a drug illegal.

What is tobacco?

Most of the tobacco we consume today is made from the dried leaves of the tobacco plant *nicotiana tabacum*, although there are many other species with a [†]long history of use. It is native to the Americas and has been used there for thousands of years. European explorers were introduced to it in the 16th century, and colonial settlers soon began cultivating it for export home. Sir Francis Drake introduced pipe-smoking to Britain in the 1570s, and the habit soon spread through English society, although tobacco remained relatively rare and expensive. King Philip II of Spain started producing cigars in Seville in 1614, and cigarettes were invented by beggars who would collect discarded cigar butts and roll the leftover tobacco in thin strips of paper. The French court's practice of sniffing snus (snuff) was brought back to Britain by Charles II, and this became the aristocrats' favourite way of taking tobacco, while the lower orders smoked it in pipes.

Ready-made cigarettes were invented in Turkey, and became popular with British soldiers when they were fighting alongside Turks during the Crimean War. These were hand-manufactured initially, but they suddenly became much cheaper in the 1880s with the invention of automatic cigarette-rolling machines. The inclusion of millions of cigarettes in soldiers' rations in the First and Second World Wars led to huge increases in the number of people addicted to tobacco. Since the 1970s, Western governments have been adopting public-health measures to reduce the social costs of tobacco and have seen a substantial drop in the number of smokers. However, in much of the rest of the world smoking is still on the rise, with devastating effects. The WHO has estimated that [†]tobacco will account for 10% of all deaths worldwide by 2015.

What are tobacco's harms and benefits?

Tobacco smoke is highly toxic. It contains [†]at least 60 chemicals known or suspected to cause cancer in humans, including arsenic, benzene and lead, as well as carbon monoxide, which damages the heart and blood vessels. Smoking carries a substantial risk of developing a range of lung problems, such as chronic bronchitis, emphysema and asthma, as well as a 20-fold increase in the likelihood of developing lung cancer. It constricts blood vessels, which can cause heart problems, cardiovascular disease, and stroke. This risk is often compounded by difficulties with heavy breathing, which make smokers less likely to take exercise and more likely to be overweight.

Because its intoxication effects are mild, tobacco isn't associated with violent or antisocial behaviour, although [†]smoking during pregnancy can damage the foetus by reducing its oxygen supply. Discarded matches and cigarette butts can cause fires; it's suspected that the [†]fire in King's Cross that killed 31 people in 1987 was started by a smoker's match. Because tobacco is legal, it's not associated with international crime (apart from some smuggling to evade tax) and the sale of cigarettes does generate large revenues for governments (although it creates substantial economic costs at the same time). Policy Exchange have calculated that [†]cigarette taxes raise £10 billion a year, but the cost to the economy of treating tobacco related health problems is £13.7 billion.

The longer the habit continues, the more the risks increase, particularly after the age of 30, as the body becomes less able to repair itself. David Spiegelhalter has calculated that [†]each cigarette takes 11 minutes off your total lifespan, based on the fact that a 30 year old smoker of 30 cigarettes a day will die on average at 69, ten years younger than someone who never smoked.

Second-hand smoke is also dangerous. It's [†]classified as a carcinogen by the WHO, and given a "class A" rating by the USA Environmental Protection Agency, in the same carcinogenic class as asbestos and arsenic. A [†]review by the UK Scientific Committee on Tobacco and Health in 2004 found that exposure to second-hand smoke contributes to medical conditions such as lung cancer, heart disease, asthma attacks and reduced lung function. Two years later, [†]the US Surgeon General reiterated these findings, emphasising that children are particularly at risk, and may suffer ear problems, acute respiratory infections, more severe asthma, slower lung growth, and an increased risk of Sudden Infant Death Syndrome ("cot death"). Although the risks are much lower than for those who smoke themselves, second-hand smoke is still responsible for [†]600,000 deaths a year worldwide, 11,000 of those in the UK.

Although it's questionable whether tobacco has any health benefits at all, there is some evidence that in later life it may reduce the risks of Parkinson's disease. While tobacco was used as a medicine for thousands of years by indigenous cultures in the Americas, their patterns of use were very different to those of today's cigarette-smokers. Peace-pipe ceremonies were highly ritualised and relatively rare, participation was usually limited to certain people (such as chiefs, medicine men and patients), and the smoke was "tasted" rather than inhaled. These factors [†]protected the users from becoming addicted to tobacco and from the carcinogenic effects of the drug. Tobacco's role in peace-pipe ceremonies was largely symbolic, carrying the thoughts and prayers of the participants towards heaven in the smoke it produced. Tobacco in Native American ceremonies is about as close to modern cigarette smoking as the consumption of wine in the Christian communion is to binge drinking.

Because of tobacco's sacred status in the Americas, when tobacco was first brought to Europe it was [†]treated as a cure-all for everything from tetanus to migraine although in fact smoking is far more harmful than beneficial. Research is ongoing as to whether isolated components of tobacco, which can be consumed in safer ways than smoking, might have some medicinal value. A lot of research has looked at nicotine, particularly because a very high proportion of people with schizophrenia smoke, and [†]it's thought that nicotine has anti-psychotic and cognition-impairing properties and may be protective in low doses. New types of nicotinergic anti-psychotics are currently being studied which don't contain nicotine but act on the same receptors. However, while some ingredients may have some therapeutic value, tobacco leaves in their natural form contain so much tar and so many carcinogenic chemicals that they would have to be *extremely* beneficial to be worth the risks, and there is no evidence that they are. Figure 11.1 shows some of the harms of smoking, compared with those of cocaine use.

	Cocaine [†](700,000 users)	Tobacco [†](7 million users)
Deaths per year	Medium – [†]about 250 in England and Wales in 2010	Very high – [†]about 100,000 in the UK a year
Physical damage	Medium – [†]about 800 non-fatal poisonings, some other heart damage	Very high – [†]1.5 million hospital admissions for tobacco-related disease every year
Psychological damage	Cocaine psychosis is rare but can occur in heavy users	None
Dependence	Medium – [†]about 12,000 people in treatment for cocaine addiction in 2007/8	Very high – [†]basically all 7 million smokers addicted
Loss of tangibles and relation-ships	Some – [†]can cause poverty, risk-taking, anti-social behaviour	Very low
Economic cost	Low – hard to estimate but [†]not more than £50 million a year	Very high – [†]£13 billion a year
International damage	Very high – [†]40,000 murders in Mexico, violence in Colombia, rainforest destruction	Medium – [†]deforestation, fertilisers deplete soil, farmers are exploited

Table 11.1: A comparison of the harms of tobacco with the harms of cocaine, in the UK.

Tobacco does release dopamine in the brain, and so creates sensations of pleasure, but this effect is very mild compared with other stimulants, even for people who are genetically predisposed to enjoy the drug more than others. Most of the pleasure of smoking is due to the social context

Drugs – without the hot air, David Nutt

and the relief of addictive cravings. Smoking is a sociable activity, and it's acceptable to ask for cigarettes, lighters or rolling papers, even from strangers; smokers also tend to have a strong sense of group identity and create social bonds while consuming cigarettes. While these benefits are real, they could equally be generated through other activities that pose lower health risks to the individual and those who passively inhale their smoke. Ultimately, what drives most habitual smokers to use the drug repeatedly are the cravings produced by their nicotine addiction; they may say that they find smoking relaxing and enjoyable but a large part of these pleasures is the relief of no longer being in nicotine withdrawal.

How do we know that smoking causes lung cancer?

As long ago as 1604, King James I of England described smoking as a [†]"custom loathsome to the eye, hateful to the nose, harmful to the brain [and] dangerous to the lungs". In the late 1700s, a London doctor noted [†]a link between using snuff and cancers of the nose, and by the [†]1850s the health effects of tobacco were being debated by medical professionals in the *Lancet*. The first strong evidence of a [†]link between lung cancer and tobacco-smoking was published in 1912, and over the next four decades the evidence mounted. When the results of [†]Richard Doll's study of 40,000 doctors over a period of 20 years was published in the 1950s, showing a 20-fold increase in the likelihood of developing lung cancer among smokers, a causal relationship seemed incontrovertible.

At first, tobacco companies took a relatively subtle approach towards the growing evidence that they were marketing a lethal drug. They advertised directly to doctors with claims that their cigarettes were less harmful than other brands, and to the public with slogans like [†]"More doctors smoke Camels than any other cigarette", to associate smoking and good health. Doll's initial research was worrying, but the industry hoped that the public wouldn't really pay much attention to a statistical study. Then in 1953, Dr. Ernst Wynder published a paper showing that [†]mice that were painted with tobacco tar developed tumours, proving that tobacco tar was carcinogenic. This was a much simpler sort of experiment to communicate to the public, and was widely reported in the press. Within the industry this wave of negative publicity was termed the "1954 emergency", and led to them developing one of the most successful PR campaigns in history.

Within weeks, the PR company hired by "big tobacco" had designed a strategy that has become a blueprint for other powerful industries. Rather than try to disprove the evidence (which would have been impossible), they focused on trying to make the link seem less certain. As long as people thought that the issue was still scientific "controversy" rather than "consensus", and other hypotheses were seen as probable, action would be delayed, and in that delay they could continue to sell large numbers of cigarettes. They began with an advert entitled [†]*A Frank Statement to Cigarette Smokers*, which appeared in 448 daily newspapers on January 4, 1954, reaching an estimated 43 million Americans. Its essential claims were that:

- Medical research of recent years indicates many possible causes of lung cancer.
- There is no agreement among the authorities regarding what the cause is.
- There is no proof that cigarette smoking is one of the causes.
- Statistics purporting to link cigarette smoke with the disease could apply with equal force to any one of many other aspects of modern life. Indeed the validity of the statistics themselves is questioned by numerous scientists.

The advertisement continued saying that they were taking the issue seriously, and were setting up a Tobacco Industry Research Committee (TIRC), to be headed by a scientist of "unimpeachable integrity and national repute" to examine the health effects of their product. In April of that year, the TIRC produced an 18-page booklet called *A Scientific Perspective on the Cigarette Controversy*, which compiled all the inconclusive or contrary results they could find about the relationship between tobacco and harms to human health. This booklet was mailed to over 200,000 doctors, politicians and journalists.

What the tobacco industry was exploiting was the fact that it's difficult

Drugs – without the hot air, David Nutt

to prove a cause and effect relationship conclusively. Just because two events have a correlation doesn't necessarily mean that one has caused the other. [†]A might have caused B, or B might have caused A, or they might both have been caused by C, a third factor that might not be immediately obvious from just looking at A and B. And even when you have proved that A and B are correlated, and that A causes B rather than the other way round, you still have to identify a mechanism. As we saw with cannabis and schizophrenia, there can be lots of confounding factors that make a definitive answer hard to come by.

In fact, the research on tobacco and lung cancer *did* prove a causal relationship. Richard Doll's study followed a huge sample of doctors over a long time period, during which some did not smoke at all, some gave up, and some continued smoking. He had a control sample – those who didn't smoke – and examples of people smoking for different periods of time, so he could see whether the risks increased the longer people smoked. The association between smoking and lung cancer was incredibly strong, about 20 times stronger than the association between not smoking and lung cancer. Wynder's mouse study had demonstrated that tobacco caused cancer, so they also had a mechanism. Doll's findings were similar to most of the other research that had been done on the subject, and have been repeated many times since, whereas the research results that the TIRC quoted in their booklet were anomalous. There are many areas of uncertainty in drug science, but the relationship between tobacco and lung cancer is not one of them.

Why is smoking so addictive?

About a fifth of adults in Britain smoke. Of these, [†]75% want to quit and 79% have tried and failed in the past. What is it about tobacco that makes it so difficult to give up? It's partly the substance itself. Nicotine is an addictive drug that leads to rapid and marked withdrawal reactions when people try to quit; these withdrawal reactions are felt by many smokers every morning, leading to the first cigarette of the day. Also, tobacco smoke contains substances that block the important brain enzyme monoamine oxidase (MAO) which can itself cause dependence. (The bright areas in the PET images in Figure 11.1 show the prevalence of MAO in a non-smoker's brain, and a smoker's.). This breaks down dopamine, so if the enzyme is blocked, levels of dopamine are increased, leading to an improved mood. In withdrawal, dopamine levels fall, and depression can result. So tobacco smoking has two components, both of which contribute to its addictiveness.

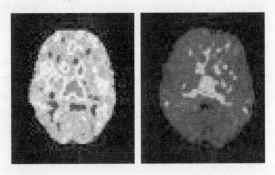

Figure 11.1: PET images of a non-smoker's brain (left) compared with a smoker's (right). The bright areas show the prevalence of the important brain enzyme monoamine oxidase (MAO).

The route of use plays a role as well. Cigarettes are second only to the hypodermic syringe in efficiency of drug delivery – smoking delivers the drug into the brain nearly as fast as injecting. Cigarettes are portable and convenient, and fit a five-minute break perfectly. In contrast, when tobacco or nicotine is consumed in forms that reach the brain more slowly, such as snuff, gum or patches, it is far less addictive. We rated tobacco the third most dependence-forming drug, after heroin and crack cocaine: 40% of people who start to smoke become addicted.

In my clinical work, I've come across people who've had to have both legs amputated after developing peripheral arterial disease from smoking. This is a terrifying example of the power of addiction, because, unlike having lung cancer, they would have got better if they'd stopped. Not being able to quit even after you've lost a leg, and continuing to

Drugs – without the hot air, David Nutt

smoke until your second leg has to be removed, shows just how powerful the drive to smoke can be.

Once addicted, a smoker will get a hit with every cigarette, and get uncomfortable withdrawal sensations in between. There are genetic vulnerabilities to tobacco dependence, some of which are related to how quickly it clears from the body: the faster you process nicotine the more likely you are to want to go back for another hit.

But it's also the social context of smoking and that makes it so difficult to give up. Many people will recall their first ecstasy pill or spliff as highly enjoyable experiences, perhaps even life-altering ones. Almost no-one enjoys their first cigarette, and it's only because popular culture is saturated with positive images of people smoking and because friends encourage it that anyone smokes a second cigarette. Tobacco is legal, freely available apart from the age restriction, and although we no longer have public advertising, still films and TV constantly associate the smoking habit with youth, attractiveness and being "cool".

Any addict will experience powerful cravings which can be triggered by the environments and social groups they associate with taking the drug. For smokers, the temptation is there every time they walk into a newsagent, see images of people enjoying cigarettes, or pass someone else smoking. Part of the aim of public-health measures like smoking bans has been to reduce these triggers: if smoking is made more inconvenient, and ex-smokers don't have to sit in smoky places, it makes it easier to fight the cravings. There's some evidence that smoking bans can help prevent people from taking up the habit in the first place. A study in 2001 of teenagers in Massachusetts found that, although there wasn't much difference in the numbers who experimented with cigarettes, they were [†]35% less likely to be habitual smokers in towns that had smoking bans. Public-health measures have also reduced smoking amongst teenagers in the UK. [†]In 1991, the number of 11–15 year olds who smoked was 16%; by 2005 this had dropped to 5%.

Public-health responses and industry resistance

By the early 1960s, it had become clear that tobacco is a highly addictive drug with serious health consequences for the millions of people hooked on it, and is the biggest cause of preventable death in the developed world. Once this was recognised as a public-health crisis, several public-health measures were introduced to reduce the harms of tobacco. The first step was to control the content of advertisements. Bizarre as it seems today, cigarette advertising in the 1940s and 50s often featured doctors making claims about the health benefits of cigarettes, at least in comparison to rival brands. Regulations led to tougher rules on where adverts could be placed (for example, not within sight of schools), disallowing sponsorship of sporting events, and eventually to an outright ban on any public advertising at all.

Restrictions limited smoking to dedicated places, and banned it completely where this was impractical, such as in planes or hospitals. Smoking in the workplace became less and less common, although it wasn't completely outlawed in the UK until the 2007 ban came into force. In some countries it's also banned in outdoor public areas like parks and beaches. Specific services for tobacco addicts were set up, such as the NHS helpline for smokers, and information about nicotine replacement therapies and other treatments started to be advertised in hospitals and GP surgeries.

Warning labels were introduced on cigarette packets across the EU in 2003, with pictures of cancer-riddled lungs and other graphic images appearing alongside them in the UK in 2007. These seem to have been reasonably effective: a survey in 2008 found that [†]30% of current smokers said the warnings helped them smoke less. 2011 saw the announcement of a new policy that will [†]require shops and newsagents to put cigarette packets "under the counter" rather than on display behind the cashier. (Australia leads the world here, and soon will require plain packets for all cigarettes.) It's hoped that making cigarettes less visible will reduce the temptation for people to make casual purchases of cigarettes as a result of nicotine cravings triggered by seeing the packets. Cigarettes in

Drugs – without the hot air, David Nutt

vending machines were banned from October 2011; this is particularly important because it removes an easy way for young people to bypass the age restriction on purchase.

At every step of the way, the tobacco industry has resisted these measures. Part of the strategy has been misinformation, deliberately spreading doubt and uncertainty about the validity of the science that shows their drug causes harm or is addictive. Another tack has been to discredit the public-health measures themselves, arguing that these are ineffective or punitive. They've suggested alternative measures, such as ventilation in place of smoking bans, claiming that they're just as effective, although [†]independent research has shown otherwise. The tobacco industry has supported institutes and research centres to conduct scientific studies that disagree with the majority of the evidence about tobacco harms. As it has become clear that industrialised countries are going to continue to restrict the sale and use of tobacco, the industry has aggressively targeted developing nations. [†]Within a few decades, 80% of tobacco related deaths will occur in the developing world.

The tobacco industry's most successful ploy, however, was to switch from promoting cigarettes as a sign of health, adulthood and responsibility, to promoting smoking as a desirable habit precisely because it is risky and subversive. This allowed them to tap two new markets: the rebellious youth culture that developed in the 1960s, and women. Freud's nephew Edward Bernays, who is often called "the father of PR", devised a stunt in 1929 in which beautiful women were hired to appear at New York's Easter Parade, smoking and holding banners calling their cigarette a "torch of liberty". The [†]association between female emancipation and smoking has had a positive result on tobacco companies profits pretty much everywhere it's been tried, and though male smokers still outnumber female smokers, the proportion of women is rising, with a corresponding rise in health problems. Official statistics show that [†]in 2006–8 lung cancer caused more deaths in women than breast cancer, almost all of these deaths due to smoking. Since the 1950s there has been a [†]600% increase in women's death rates for lung cancer.

Like the alcohol industry, for a long time tobacco companies argued that they didn't need statutory regulation and that voluntary codes were enough to improve their behaviour and reduce harm. The attitude within governments has fortunately changed on this score, and although there's still more to be done to reduce the influence of the tobacco industry, at least making laws to control its reach is recognised as the most effective way to improve public health. This change in attitude has taken a long time, for (as with alcohol) the industry has had a big ace up its sleeve in terms of influencing policymakers: many of the people making decisions about how tobacco should be regulated have themselves been addicted. Smoking wasn't even recognised as an addiction in the United States until 1989 – before that it was referred to as a "habituation", downplaying how difficult it was for many people to stop. The fact that many politicians were smokers themselves undoubtedly played a role in this sort of thinking.

Consequences of the UK smoking ban

Did the UK 2007 smoking ban work? It's important to evaluate any policy to determine whether it's been effective in achieving its aims, and whether it's had any unintended consequences. The main aim of the ban was to protect people from the effects of second-hand smoke; given that [†]compliance was above 98%, it undoubtedly achieved this. A study of bar workers measured the amount of cotinine (a byproduct of nicotine that gives the best measure of exposure to tobacco smoke) present in their saliva, and found it had [†]dropped by 76% after the ban was brought in.

There were some immediate and obvious health benefits to the change. [†]Air quality in bars, which had previously been at "unhealthy" levels, dramatically improved, encouraging non-smokers into them. It also benefited people with lung conditions: [†]a third said it helped keep them out of hospital. There was also a [†]2.4% reduction in heart attacks in England in the 12 months following the ban, although we don't know if this was related to lower levels of passive smoking or direct smoking, as there was also a marked drop in cigarette sales. A year after the ban, it was

Drugs – without the hot air, David Nutt

estimated that [†]2 billion fewer cigarettes had been smoked in the period June 2007–2008, compared with the year June 2006–2007. This has partly been attributed to the ban, although raising the age of sale to 18 and increasing tax also helped to reduce demand.

Whether the ban achieved one of its secondary aims – to reduce the environmental triggers and help people give up their addiction – is more uncertain. In the year following the ban, there was a [†]22% increase in demand for NHS stop-smoking services, although this may have just been a short-term gain. Another study found that [†]prescriptions for anti-smoking drugs increased by 6.4% in the nine months before the ban, but fell by 6.4% in the nine months after. It's possible that the publicity around the change may have influenced people who already wanted to quit, but once they had stopped we were left with a hard-core of smokers with little motivation to quit. These may have found access to outdoor smoking areas and contact with other people who smoke more influential than the fact they could no longer smoke inside.

We've seen how easy it is for well-intentioned policies to end up having perverse effects when they don't take into account the real-world situation in which they're going to be implemented, but so far predictions about negative consequences of the ban have not been borne out. [†]MP John Reid opposed the bill, saying that it would increase smoking in the home, when in fact there was a rise in the number of families *not* allowing smoking at home, [†]from 61% in 2006 to 67% in 2008. Nor was there mass civil disobedience by frustrated smokers, nor widespread non-compliance by proprietors, and public support has remained steady at about 76%. Apart from a few isolated cases of people openly refusing to accept the ban, compliance has been high, although some places do hold after-hours smoke-ins, which tend to be tolerated by councils and police in the same way that alcohol lock-ins are. The claims by sites like [†]Opposingthe-UK-smokingban.org that smokers have been murdered and violently attacked for their habit since the ban don't seem to have any basis in reality; in fact, the most [†]well-known incident of "smoke rage" was aimed at a non-smoker, when a restaurant owner in Turkey was killed in 2009 after trying to enforce the smoking ban which had just been implemented there.

Some businesses have suffered loss of revenue, although this was a predictable consequence rather than a perverse one. [†]175 million fewer pints were sold in pubs between July 2007 and April 2008 than in the year before (which would actually mark an improvement to the nation's health if it hadn't in all likelihood been replaced with drinking cut-price supermarket alcohol at home). The solution to the hospitality trade's problems, as we said in chapter 6 on alcohol, is not to reintroduce smoking, but to encourage people back into the pub by removing the price differential betwen off-licence and pub. The improved air quality does seem to have encouraged non-smokers to spend more time at their local: in an opinion survey a year after the ban, [†]11% of people said they were now spending less time in the pub, but 13% said they were going there more, partly because it was now a more pleasant place to be.

Freedom and choice

Many people objected to the smoking ban on the grounds that it violated their freedom to choose to smoke. This point about "freedom" is worth thinking about, because a lot of arguments made about the regulation of drugs come from a libertarian stance that emphasises our right to be free from the influence of others. Libertarians are economically right-wing, and think that the state shouldn't interfere with markets or people's freedom to make choices for themselves. In the UK, the most prominent libertarian party is the UK Independence Party, and although they are best known for being anti-EU they also have policies on decriminalising drugs, arguing that the state shouldn't decide what's best for individuals.

It's important to make clear how my position differs from theirs. I think our goal should be to reduce the harm done by drugs, and because sending people to prison causes more harm than drugs, it is an ineffective and unjust policy. That's not the same as thinking that people should be free to do just what they like. I do believe that restricting people's rights to engage in *all* risky activities would be disproportionate and unfair – there would be a general outcry if we tried to ban horse riding, for example. But when considering the issue of free choice about the drugs we

Drugs – without the hot air, David Nutt

consume we have to bear three things in mind.

Firstly, you are only free to choose if you have correct information, and this means being free from false or misleading presentations of the benefits and risks of an activity. Advertising is always going to emphasise benefits and obscure harms, and so it confounds our freedom to choose. When tobacco advertising was still permitted, the tobacco industry used images of youth, health, beauty and desirability to imply that this is what the outcome of using cigarettes would be, when the truth is that half of all smokers will end their days dying of a smoking-related disease. Today, branded packaging uses light colours, pictures of filters, and words like "mild" to give the impression that these cigarettes will be healthier, when research shows that †the harm they cause is the same as any other brands. The groundwork done by popular culture to glamorise drug-taking is particularly notable with cigarettes, since for most people their initial experiences are unpleasant – they have to be motivated by positive ideas of what smoking means in order to come to enjoy it. Since documents used during tobacco trials in the 1990s were made public, we have huge amounts of proof of the ways in which †the industry distorted evidence, misled customers, and lied publicly about the dangers of their product. Protecting people's freedom to choose requires providing them with objective facts and ensuring they aren't given false information.

Secondly, you can't make a free choice if you're an addict. This is not to say that addicts can't get "clean", but that addiction changes our brains and impairs our judgement, so an addict's choice of whether or not to smoke a cigarette is completely different to the choice a non-addict makes. Your first 100 cigarettes might be freely chosen, but once your brain has adapted to the drug, your desire to have your 101st is mostly driven by the unpleasantness of nicotine withdrawal. Protecting people's freedom to choose must include taking steps to avoid addiction.

And thirdly, while libertarians emphasise their right to live without being influenced by others, drug-taking isn't an isolated, personal matter. Your freedom to have a drink and get in your car directly affects other people's freedom to be safe on the road, just as your freedom to have a cigarette where you like affects other people's freedom to choose whether or not to be exposed to your smoke. An important part of this impact on other people is the costs that are covered by public services. I believe, as the majority of people in the UK do, that free public health-care (ie the NHS) benefits everybody, and that nobody should remain untreated even if their illness is partly self-inflicted. Tobacco addicts are also taxpayers, and while banning smoking in public places restricts them as smokers, it increases their freedom as taxpayers by releasing money from treating tobacco-related illnesses.

In the end, even some of the most staunch proponents of this particular idea of freedom have found their own "free choices" have had consequences which have led them to rely on society for support. One of the 20th century's most famous libertarians, Ayn Rand, spent a lifetime arguing that state interference was immoral, but ended her life on Medicare being treated for smoking-related lung cancer.

Conclusion

Smoking was banned in public places because tobacco is harmful, both to smokers and to those exposed to second-hand smoke. Around half of those who use tobacco regularly will die of a tobacco related disease; and around [†]11,000 people a year die in the UK from the effects of passive smoking, out of a total of 80,000 tobacco-related deaths [†](Figure 11.2).

Smoking is extremely addictive, and many people find it very difficult to give up, even when they know it's harming them and others around them. When people in poorer countries take up the habit, where the risks are compounded by poor diets, by not having access to healthcare, and by high levels of pollution, the likelihood of tobacco causing illness is even higher. At current trends, we will have allowed tobacco to [†]kill a billion people by 2030.

Criminalisation would create a huge black market, and would probably face so much non-compliance that it would be unenforceable. It would also deprive governments of tax revenue (which covers some of the costs of treating tobacco-related diseases), and we would lose our ability to reclaim some of the industry's enormous profits. Instead of

Drugs – without the hot air, David Nutt

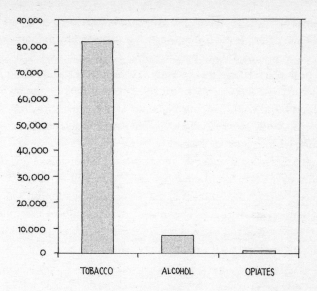

Figure 11.2: Annual deaths in the UK due to different drugs.

seeing this as a moral issue to be punished through the criminal justice system, governments have recognised that tobacco addiction is a public-health crisis, to be dealt with through education, giving support to drug users, restricting availability, raising prices, and controlling the companies that make money out of getting people hooked.

Our efforts to minimise the harms done by tobacco show us both the dangers of allowing a drug to be openly marketed in society, and some of the most effective steps we can take to reduce the harms which have resulted.

Notes

Page

192   Individuals who broke the ban would face a £50 fine, while owners could be charged £2,500 for failing to prevent smoking on their premises• *A quick guide to the smokefree law*, Smokefree England/Department of Health, URL-88, 2008

192   three quarters of adults supported the legislation• As above.

193   40% in 1978 to about 20% today• *Smoking ban has saved 40,000 lives*, Jeremy Laurence, URL-89, June 30th 2008

193   long history of use• *Exotic Substances: in introduction and global spread of tobacco, coffee, cocoa, tea and distilled liquor, sixteenth to eighteenth centuries*, Rudi Matthee, in Drugs and Narcotics in History, Cambridge University Press, 1995

194   tobacco will account for 10% of all deaths worldwide by 2015•Fact sheet, WHO, URL-90, accessed December 7th 2011

194   at least 60 chemicals known or suspected to cause cancer in humans• *The Tobacco Atlas*, WHO, URL-91, accessed December 10th 2011

194   smoking during pregnancy can damage the foetus• *The Tobacco Atlas*, WHO, URL-91, accessed December 10th 2011

194   fire in King's Cross that killed 31 people in 1987 was started by a smoker's match• *On this day*, BBC, URL-92, 18th November 1987

194   cigarette taxes raise £10 billion a year, but the cost to the economy of treating tobacco related health problems is £13.7 billion• *Cough Up*, Policy Exchange, URL-42, March 18th 2010

194   each cigarette takes 11 minutes off your total lifespan• *Time for a smoke? One cigarette reduces your life by 11 minutes*, Mary Shaw, Richard Mitchell and Danny Dorling, British Medical Journal 320(7226), January 1st 2000

195   classified as a carcinogen by the WHO• *A quick guide to the smokefree law*, Smokefree England/Department of Health, URL-88, 2008

195   review by the UK Scientific Committee on Tobacco and Health in 2004• *Second hand smoke: a review of evidence since 1998*, Scientific Committee on Tobacco and Health, URL-93, November 2004

195   the US Surgeon General reiterated these findings• *The health consequences of involuntary exposure to tobacco smoke: a report of the surgeon general*, URL-94, June 27th 2006

195   600,000 deaths a year worldwide, 11,000 of those in the UK•Fact sheet, WHO URL-90, accessed December 7th 2011

195 protected the users from becoming addicted to tobacco• *Tobacco use by Native Americans: sacred smoke and silent killer*, Joseph Winter (ed.), University of Oklahoma Press, 2000

195 treated as a cure-all for everything from tetanus to migraine• *Medicinal uses of tobacco in history*, Anne Charlton, Journal of the Royal Society of Medicine 97 (6), June 2004

196 it's thought that nicotine has anti-psychotic and cognition-impairing properties• *A review of the effects of nicotine on schizophrenia and antipsychotic medications*, Edward Lyon, Psychiatric Services, October 1st 1999

196 (700,000 users)• *Drug Misuse Declared: Findings from the 2010/11 British Crime Survey*, Office of National Statistics, URL-108, July 2011

196 (7 million users)• *Statistics on Smoking: England 2011*, NHS the Information Centre, URL-109, 2011

196 about 250 in England and Wales in 2010• *National Programme on Substance Abuse Deaths*, International Centre for Drug Policy, 2010

196 about 100,000 in the UK a year• extrapolated from the figure of 81,700 in England, from *Statistics on Smoking: England 2011*, NHS the Information Centre, URL-109, 2011

196 about 800 non-fatal poisonings, some other heart damage• *The Cocaine Trade*, House of Commons Home Affairs Committee, URL-110, February 23rd 2010

196 1.5 million hospital admissions for tobacco-related disease every year• *Statistics on Smoking: England 2011*, NHS the Information Centre, URL-109, 2011

196 about 12,000 people in treatment for cocaine addiction in 2007/8• *The Cocaine Trade*, House of Commons Home Affairs Committee, URL-110, February 23rd 2010

196 basically all 7 million smokers addicted• This is because the definition of being a "smoker" in most surveys means smoking sufficiently frequently for nicotine addiction to have taken place.

196 can cause poverty, risk-taking, anti-social behaviour• *The Cocaine Trade*, House of Commons Home Affairs Committee, URL-110, February 23rd 2010

196 not more than £50 million a year• Nicola Singleton, Rosemary Murray and Louise Tinsley, Home Office, URL-111, 2006. In this report, Class A drug use in 2003/4 was estimated to be around £15.4bn, of which problematic opiate and crack cocaine use accounted for 99% (£15.3bn). This means that the cost of all other Class A drug use totalled £100m. Assuming that (at the

very most) cocaine powder accounted for half of these costs, it still won't exceed £50m a year.

196 £13 billion a year• *Cough Up*, Policy Exchange, URL-42, March 18th 2010

196 40,000 murders in Mexico, violence in Colombia, rainforest destruction• See chapter 10.

196 deforestation, fertilisers deplete soil, farmers are exploited• *Growing Tobacco*, WHO Tobacco Atlas, URL-112, accessed December 10th 2011

197 "custom loathsome to the eye, hateful to the nose, harmful to the brain [and] dangerous to the lungs"• *A Counterblast to Tobacco*, King James I, URL-95, 1604

197 a link between using snuff and cancers of the nose• *Cautions against the immoderate use of snuff*, John Hill, printed for R. Baldwin and J. Jackson, 1761

197 1850s the health effects of tobacco were being debated by medical professionals in the *Lancet*• *The Great Tobacco Question: is Smoking Injurious to Health?*, Lancet, 1856

197 link between lung cancer and tobacco-smoking was published in 1912• *Primary malignant growth of the lung and bronchii*, Isaac Adler, Longmans, Green, 1912

197 Richard Doll's study of 40,000 doctors over a period of 20 years was published in the 1950s• *British doctors study*, Richard Doll, British Medical Journal, 1950

197 "More doctors smoke Camels than any other cigarette"• original advert, Camel cigarettes, URL-96, 1949

197 mice that were painted with tobacco tar developed tumours• *Tobacco smoking as a possible aetiological factor in bronchiogenic carcinoma: a study of 684 proven cases*, Wynder, Journal of the American Medical Association, 1950

198 *A Frank Statement to Cigarette Smokers*• Legacy Tobacco Documents Library, URL-97, 1954

199 A might have caused B, or B might have caused A, or they might both have been caused by C, a third factor that might not be immediately obvious from just looking at A and B.• A simple example of a flawed association is between shoe-size (A) and reading ability (B). If you survey shoe-size and reading ability in a large population, there is a very strong correlation. However, large shoe-size does *not* cause a person to be good at reading; in fact, shoe-size and reading-ability are more accurately correlated with a third factor, age (C) – adults have bigger feet than children, and many children are still just learning to read.

A less trivial example is the current investigation between taking cannabis (A) and schizophrenia (B); both may be linked to a genetic variation (C) that predisposes a person both to take cannabis and to suffer from schizophrenia.

199 75% want to quit and 79% have tried and failed in the past• *A quick guide to the smokefree law*, Smokefree England/Department of Health, URL-88, 2008

201 35% less likely to be habitual smokers in towns that had smoking bans• *Local Restaurant Smoking Regulations and the Adolescent Smoking Initiation Process*, Michael Siegel et al, Archives of Pediatric and Adolescent Medicine 162 (5), 2008

201 In 1991, the number of 11–15 year olds who smoked was 16%; by 2005 this had dropped to 5%• *From underwear to aircraft noise: logging 70 years of social change*, Office for National Statistics, URL-98, September 2nd 2011

202 30% of current smokers said the warnings helped them smoke less• *Survey on Tobacco Analytical Report*, European Commission, March 2009

202 require shops and newsagents to put cigarette packets "under the counter" rather than on display behind the cashier.•BBC, *Tobacco display ban reminder for supermarkets*, URL-159, December 28, 2011.

203 independent research has shown otherwise• *Dealing with the health effects of secondhand smoke*, Select Committee on Health First Report, URL-99, 2005

203 Within a few decades, 80% of tobacco related deaths will occur in the developing world•Fact sheet, WHO, URL-90, accessed December 7th 2011

203 association between female emancipation and smoking has had a positive result on tobacco companies profits• *Gender empowerment and female-to-male smoking prevalence ratios*, Sara Hitchman and Geoffrey Fong, Bulletin of the World Health Organization, URL-24, January 5th 2011. The authors quote an internal industry document from 1991: "To convince fashionable, modern, independent and self-confident women aged 20–34 that by smoking [Virginia Slims], they are making better/more complete expression of their independence."

203 in 2006–8 lung cancer caused more deaths in women than breast cancer• *Cancer incidence and mortality in the UK 2006–2008*, Office for National Statistics, URL-100, June 2011

203 600% increase in women's death rates for lung cancer• *An epidemic of smoking-related cancer and disease in women*, URL-101, August 2010.

204 compliance was above 98%• *A quick guide to the smokefree law*, Smokefree England/Department of Health, URL-88, 2008

204 dropped by 76% after the ban was brought in• *A quick guide to the smokefree law*, Smokefree England/Department of Health, URL-88, 2008

204 Air quality in bars, which had previously been at "unhealthy" levels, dramatically improved• As above.

204 a third said it helped keep them out of hospital• *Smoking ban has saved 40,000 lives*, Jeremy Laurance, URL-89, June 30th 2008

204 2.4% reduction in heart attacks• *Heart attacks fall after smoking ban*, NHS Choices, URL-102, June 9th 2010

205 2 billion fewer cigarettes had been smoked• *Smoking ban has saved 40,000 lives*, Jeremy Laurance, URL-89, June 30th 2008

205 22% increase in demand for NHS stop-smoking services• *A quick guide to the smokefree law*, Smokefree England/Department of Health, URL-88, 2008

205 prescriptions for anti-smoking drugs increased by 6.4% in the nine months before the ban, but fell by 6.4% in the nine months after• *The impact of the introduction of smoke free legislation on prescribing of stop-smoking medications in England*, Szatkowski et al, Addiction, July 27th 2011

205 MP John Reid opposed the bill• *MPs to challenge ministers veto on total smoking ban*, Patrick Wintour, the *Guardian*, December 17th 2005

205 from 61% in 2006 to 67% in 2008• *A quick guide to the smokefree law*, Smokefree England/Department of Health, URL-88, 2008

205 Opposingthe-UK-smokingban.org• describe themselves as promoting the "freedom to choose" and that their mission is "to fight against the injustice of smokers being treated as second class citizens (and to dispel the myth about Second Hand Smoke) in the UK!" URL-103.

205 well-known incident of "smoke rage" was aimed at a non-smoker, when a restaurant owner in Turkey was killed in 2009 after trying to enforce the smoking ban which had just been implemented there• *Smoking ban murder*, Reuters, URL-104, July 31st 2009

206 175 million fewer pints were sold in pubs between July 2007 and April 2008 than in the year before• *Smoking ban has saved 40,000 lives*, Jeremy Laurence, URL-89, June 30th 2008

206 11% of people said they were now spending less time in the pub, but 13% said they were going there more• *A quick guide to the smokefree law*, Smokefree England/Department of Health, URL-88, 2008

207 the harm they cause is the same as any other brands• *Why cigarette packs matter*, Ben Goldacre, URL-105, March 12th 2011

207 the industry distorted evidence, misled customers, and lied publicly about the dangers of their product• *The tobacco industry documents: an introductory handbook and resource for researchers*, Ross Mackenzie, Jeff Collin & Kelley Lee, URL-106, July 2003. This is a good introduction to Tobacco Documents Online, about 40 million pages of documents from tobacco companies and industry organisations, released after the tobacco trials of the 1990s in the USA.

208 11,000 people a year die in the UK from the effects of passive smoking• Cancer Research UK, URL-107, accessed December 10th 2011

208 (Figure 11.2).• Sources: *Smoking and drinking among adults*, 2009. Office for National Statistics; *Drug Misuse Declared: Findings from the 2010/11 British Crime Survey England and Wales*, Home Office; *Estimates of the Prevalence of Opiate Use and/or Crack Cocaine Use, 2009/10: Sweep 6 report*, The Centre for Drug Misuse Research.

208 kill a billion people by 2030• *A quick guide to the smokefree law*, Smokefree England/Department of Health, URL-88, 2008

12 Prescription drugs – Am I addicted to Valium, Doctor?

So far we have focused largely on drugs that are broadly considered "recreational", though as we've seen the line between recreational and medicinal use is not clear-cut. This chapter is about the other side of that blurred line: drugs that have been prescribed for legitimate mental and physical illnesses but which are diverted and misused, and sometimes cause addiction. We also look at some common concerns about the long-term effects of prescribed drugs such as antidepressants, and about the motivations of the pharmaceutical industry.

The problem has two main aspects: (a) people who receive medication on prescription and take too much, or become dependent, and (b) those who use them without medical direction. Both of these are called "diversion". Sometimes people use their prescription as a source of income – for example, there is a small market for old ladies selling their sleeping pills to recreational users. Although physical dependence can happen when these drugs are taken therapeutically, the psychological cravings of addiction seem to occur only when these drugs are taken in non-prescribed ways.

The most common prescription drugs that are diverted and misused are: benzodiazepines prescribed for anxiety and sleep disorders; painkillers such as codeine, morphine and oxycodone; and stimulants such as Ritalin prescribed for attention deficit hyperactivity disorder which we'll cover in chapter 13.

What are benzodiazepines and how do they work?

Benzodiazepines first appeared in the 1960s, for treating a range of physical and mental-health problems. Benzodiazepines replaced barbiturates, another sedative tranquilliser that had been around since the 1860s, and were the first wave of drugs found to be effective for severe anxiety. However, concerns that barbiturates were leading to behavioural disturbances, physical dependence, and addiction, as well as high-profile cases of barbiturate-assisted suicide like Marilyn Monroe's, led to the search for a less dangerous form of depressant medication. The first benzodiazepine, Librium, was approved for medicinal use in 1960, and diazepam followed in 1963 under the trade name Valium. Other popular "benzos" are Ativan, Xanax, Rohypnol and Mogadon, and chemists have discovered thousands more.

Benzodiazepines act by increasing the effects of whatever GABA is present, so they require GABA to be released if they are to work. As we learnt in chapter 4, GABA calms the brain, like pressing an off switch. Drugs that target GABA receptors carry a risk of overdose and death if someone takes too much and switches off essential functions, including breathing. Benzodiazepines are different to depressants such as alcohol and barbiturates, because the way benzodiazepines work on GABA receptors means that their effects can't exceed the effects of the GABA that naturally occurs in the brain. This makes them much safer in overdose: the brain can compensate by switching off GABA release and so reduce the effects of the benzodiazepine. We do produce endogenous benzodiazepines – endozapines – and though we're not entirely sure what their function is, they may have evolved to regulate anxiety. It's possible that anxiety disorders and insomnia may be due to a deficit of endozapines; if this is the case, continual, long-term replacement therapy would be appropriate, just as diabetics take insulin long-term.

What are the benefits and harms of benzodiazepines?

Medicinally, benzodiazepines are usually prescribed for anxiety disorders and for people who have trouble sleeping. About [†]14% of older people in the UK take them every night, and many use them for decades. They can help relieve muscle spasm: they are used to treat convulsive disorders like epilepsy, and are routinely given before procedures like endoscopies to reduce anxiety and prevent the formation of stressful memories. When alcoholics are in acute alcohol withdrawal, benzodiazepines are used to relieve acute agitation, tremor, seizures, and delirium tremens.

Benzodiazepines usually have few side effects at therapeutic doses, although they can sometimes cause symptoms like sedation, lightheadedness, heart palpitations and headaches. GABA is essential to memory formation, and benzodiazepines can cause mild impairment, but this in itself can be therapeutic because one of the features of anxiety and PTSD is the recurrence of powerful negative memories. If benzodiazepines do cause cognitive impairment it will diminsh once the person comes off the medication.

When taken recreationally, or at higher doses than recommended by the doctor, benzodiazepines can cause respiratory depression, and although far safer than barbiturates they're still commonly used by people committing suicide. They are especially dangerous when taken with other sedatives such as alcohol, or with other drugs that depress breathing, such as opiates. The majority of people who could strictly be defined as "addicted" to benzodiazepines are heroin addicts who take them to reduce the negative effects that occur as the heroin high wears off. Many deaths reported as heroin overdoses are actually the result of the interaction between these two drugs, frequently with alcohol involved as well.

Physical dependence

Physical dependence on benzodiazepines is common. Stopping suddenly can cause severe withdrawal symptoms and even convulsions, especially if you've used them for a long time. Even when the dose is tapered, some people still experience symptoms such as rapid heartbeat, insomnia, irritability, anxiety, weight loss and muscle cramps. However, when coming off is supervised by a doctor, these symptoms are rarely severe even in long-term users. One study found that [†]80% of the subjects, who had taken benzodiazepines for an average of 17 years to help them sleep, stopped without any trouble with a gradual reduction in dose and information about sleep hygiene.

All drugs that work on the GABA receptor have the effect of "down-regulating" it, leading to the build-up of tolerance so that over time more of the drug is required to have the same therapeutic effect. Figure 12.1 shows the different possible outcomes that might result from a course of benzodiazepine treatment for an anxiety disorder.

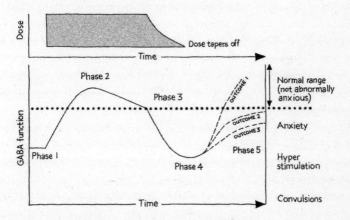

Figure 12.1: The changes in GABA function over the different phases of treating anxiety with a benzodiazepine.

- In Phase 1, the patient has abnormally-low GABA function and feels anxious all the time.
- In Phase 2, the doctor has prescribed a benzodiazepine, which improves the patient's GABA function and brings them into the normal range for anxiety (ie they'll feel anxious only when something particularly stressful or difficult is happening, rather than all the time). Over time, however, they build up tolerance to the drugs and the GABA function decreases again, but they are still OK.
- In Phase 3, the doctor tapers off their dose.
- Coming off the drugs leads to Phase 4, where withdrawal makes the patient feel even more anxious than they felt when they first

went to the doctor. However, once this period of withdrawal has passed, they will probably feel better than they did before treatment.

- In Phase 5, if the medication has been particularly successful they might experience "outcome 1", where their GABA function and levels of anxiety are now in the normal range. And even in the less successful outcomes 2 and 3, while they continue to have decreased GABA function and heightened anxiety, their condition is still less severe than before treatment.

Essentially, it seems that if you are well, you should be able to stop by tapering off your dose gradually over the course of several months, possibly switching first to Valium as it takes a long time to leave your system (around eight days) so the body has more time to adjust to the reduction of the drug in the system. If you're unwell, stopping may cause distress or withdrawal symptoms, but as these drugs are often prescribed for anxiety disorders it can be hard to know if this distress is actually a withdrawal effect, or the underlying disorder making a reappearance in the absence of medication.

Another example of how withdrawal symptoms can be confused with the disorder being treated is when this type of drug is prescribed for epilepsy. Epilepsy is characterised by seizures (characteristically, bouts of extreme muscular activity), which benzodiazepines help to control. If an epileptic stops their medication they will probably start having seizures again; these may occur alongside side-effects from coming off the drug, but aren't themselves *caused* by coming off the drug.

Panic attacks experienced by people with chronic anxiety are rather like seizures. We can see from scans that the brain's activity is abnormal, and you could think of them as seizures of the anxiety circuits (whereas epileptics experience seizures of the muscle/movement circuits). Like anxiety, epilepsy also has a long history of being misunderstood, mostly carrying heavy stigma although occasionally seen as a divine gift in some cultures. Perhaps in the future we'll understand anxiety disorders in a more sophisticated way, and be able to treat them much more effectively.

In general, although physical dependence on benzodiazepines is com-

Drugs – without the hot air, David Nutt

mon and withdrawal can sometimes be problematic, the psychological cravings that characterise addiction are extremely rare when benzodiazepines are taken as directed by the doctor. Whether it's worth risking building up tolerance and possibly suffering withdrawal symptoms, depends on individual factors – especially how ill you are and how much the benzodiazepines help you. The decision requires the same sort of weighing up of the harms and benefits as with any drug.

Antidepressants and SSRIs

Selective serotonin reuptake inhibitors (*SSRIs*) were first developed in the 1970s. They have become the most-commonly prescribed type of antidepressants worldwide in the last two decades. Common drugs of this type are citalopram (sold under the trade names Celexa and Cipramil), paroxetine (Seroxat), sertraline (Zoloft) and fluoxetine (Prozac).

SSRIs work in both depression and anxiety disorders. Depression was previously treated with tricyclic antidepressants such as amitriptyline and imipramine; although SSRIs are no more effective, [†]they have fewer side effects and almost no abuse potential. They are almost impossible to overdose on, so they are unlikely to be used to commit suicide, unlike the tricyclic antidepressant drugs which used to kill many hundreds of people per year. SSRIs work by blocking the reuptake of serotonin into its nerve terminals, so that serotonin levels in the brain slowly increase. In some people this increase in serotonin can be somewhat unpleasant, and insomnia, anxiety and restlessness commonly occur in the first few weeks of use. As a result, SSRIs are not abused, because getting used to them requires a lot of motivation. Over time these negative feelings wear off but the antidepressant effect remains, lifting the depressive mood or reducing the anxiety state. In the treatment of anxiety, medications that work on the serotonin system are an improvement on those that work on GABA, because they don't lead to a down-regulation of serotonin receptors in the way that barbiturates and benzodiazepines down-regulate GABA receptors and cause withdrawal symptoms.

Do SSRIs increase the risk of suicide?

Concerns have been raised in recent years that SSRIs might be associated with increased risk of suicide or even homicide (though the latter is so rare that it's probably impossible to prove causality). The relationship between antidepressants and suicide is complicated because, unsurprisingly, depressed people are far more likely to kill themselves than the rest of the population – about 12 times more likely if mildly or moderately depressed, and 30 times if severely depressed. There's also the well-known "energisation effect", where depressed people commit suicide after receiving treatment and seeing their symptoms improve, because at their lowest ebb they didn't have the energy or ability to plan or carry out a suicide attempt. For most people, however, receiving treatment *reduces* the risk of suicide, and this holds true with SSRIs. Indeed, the drop in suicide rates in countries like Sweden, Hungary and the USA in the past two decades is thought to be partly the result of SSRIs being more widely prescribed so there are fewer people with depression.

The first few weeks of taking SSRIs can be rather miserable in some patients, and this worsening of symptoms may make people consider killing themselves. It's very important that doctors inform the patient that these side-effects are expected and normal and will pass, and that after a few weeks the patient should feel the benefits. There does seem to be an elevated risk of suicidal ideas among adolescents, but all antidepressants have limited effectiveness on this demographic anyway, and are not recommended for under 18s. Their "clean" pharmacology – they work only on the serotonin reuptake – means that they are almost impossible to overdose on; this makes them safer than other medications, because reducing people's access to methods for killing themselves reduces the rate of suicide.

Do SSRIs cause dependence?

Most of the psychiatric disorders treated with SSRIs are long-lasting and have high rates of *relapse*, and *recurrence*. Relapse is when the first episode returns; recurrence is when a new episode of illness begins after full recovery. Over a 20-year period, almost everyone who has had one episode of depression will have another one, and the more frequently it has occurred the more likely it is to happen again – a kind of vicious cycle. There seems to be a similar pattern in some anxiety problems such as panic disorders, though others, such as PTSD, tend to be chronic. The most powerful effect of SSRIs is preventing the recurrence of these disorders so long as patients continue to take their treatment.

Unlike benzodiazepines and Ritalin, SSRIs have no street value. They give no pleasure and if anything are unpleasant at first. This makes them highly unlikely to produce the psychological cravings that characterise addiction, confirmed by the fact that animals do not self-administer them even when familiarised with them. In turn, this means medical supplies of SSRIs rarely get diverted.

To explore whether SSRIs might cause dependence (defined by physical withdrawal symptoms), we'll now examine what withdrawal means in a clinical setting.

Rebound and discontinuation

Rebound is when discontinuing the medication causes a deterioration in the condition being treated. Examples are when people with hypertension have an increase in blood pressure when they stop taking clonidine, and women becoming more fertile when they stop taking the contraceptive pill. Sometimes the deterioration can be so great that the patient's condition is worse than before they started treatment; this is called "overshoot". This can be very distressing, and in the case of conditions like epilepsy, potentially lethal.

In the treatment of depression with SSRIs, rebound is *less* likely the longer the patient has been taking them. This makes them different to benzodiazepines, which are *more* likely to cause problems if someone has been taking them for a long time. An analogy would be in the treatment of diabetes – benzodiazepines are like insulin, maintaining the person but not dealing with the underlying disorders, while SSRIs are more like dietary treatment, which takes longer to work but has more profound and long-lasting effects.

Stopping taking SSRIs can cause a discontinuation syndrome (which is different from withdrawal, because in discontinuation the symptoms are different from the underlying illness). The discontinuation syndrome is characterised by nausea, dizziness, lethargy, headache and an influenza-like feeling; these symptoms are definitely caused by the lack of drugs because they're fully reversed with another dose. If left untreated they tend to peak after 2 to 5 days, and then decay quickly over a few more days, although occasionally they can last several weeks. It may be that people with certain personality traits are more prone than others to experiencing these symptoms. It's extremely rare, however, for someone to find themselves unable come off SSRIs at all.

Painkillers

Common painkillers that can be subject to abuse include paracetamol, aspirin, ibuprofen, and codeine and other opiates such as morphine. Obviously, the more powerful the drug, the more likely someone is to become physically dependent on it, but abuse may be less common because there are stricter controls on how it is made available. Anything stronger than codeine is not available over the counter, and even codeine without a prescription can be bought in very low strength varieties only.

As with other therapeutic drugs, the medical context can protect people against addiction to painkillers, even if they have withdrawal symptoms when they stop taking them. For example, when people in chronic pain are given morphine, doctors are often concerned that they'll get addicted, but it's unusual for the patients to experience psychological cravings as they don't associate morphine with pleasure. In general, people around the world are probably under-treated with painkillers rather than over-treated, and experience great suffering as a result. Many countries have such strict controls on morphine that cancer patients and the terminally ill are left to die in agony. Heroin is even more strictly controlled, and the USA and German medical systems never use it at all, even though it's the most effective drug for extreme pain.

The physical harms of milder painkillers are well known. Aspirin is toxic to the stomach and can cause ulcers, while paracetamol is toxic to the liver. Using codeine and other painkillers incorrectly can actually sensitise people to pain, causing analgesic-induced headaches. "Incorrect use" might mean taking too much of the painkiller, or taking it too often, which might also lead to addiction, but the headaches can happen even if the patient isn't addicted. These should stop once the patient comes off the medication.

There is a difficult balance to be struck between protecting people from addiction and being able to treat them effectively. In the USA, where strong painkillers like oxycodone are much more readily accessible, patients do sometimes misuse them, and there is also a problem with drugs being diverted to family and friends who then become dependent or addicted. In the UK the medical profession is generally so reluctant to dispense painkillers that diversion of this sort isn't much of a problem, but it does mean that some people with chronic pain suffer unnecessarily. In fact, concerns about misuse of the active ingredients in medicines can lead to them being made ineffective: for example, we've removed the codeine from cough medicine out of concern that people might take too much, and now many don't work to suppress coughing at all!

The pharmaceutical industry and science

Most new medications are produced by a handful of pharmaceuticals companies, known colloquially as "big Pharma". The pharmaceutical industry comes under a lot of criticism, and many people worry about the sort of drugs it produces. The main concern seems to be that the medications sold are ineffective, unnecessary or will have unpleasant side-effects. While there are certainly examples of harmful drugs having been approved in the past (for example, when thalidomide was given to pregnant women and the children were born with birth defects), today the pharmaceutical industry is one of the most heavily-regulated in the world and the process for getting a drug approved is extremely rigorous. This process has a number of stages:

- The company chooses a target drug to investigate.
- They run toxicology tests on animals to determine its safety ratio,

its longer-term effects, and whether it's addictive.

- They then move on to studies on healthy volunteer human subjects to establish correct dosage.
- Clinical trials begin.
- After two positive trials, the company can apply for marketing authorisation.

Clinical trials are designed to be as transparent as possible. Patients (suffering from the illness the drug is designed to treat) are entered into the trial by their doctor. Half the trial subjects are randomly assigned to be given the new drug, and the other half to be given a placebo (or an existing treatment, depending on the illness). The patients don't know whether they are being given the new drug or the placebo, so the trial is *blind*. In fact, normally even the doctor doesn't know which medication their patient is taking, and then the trial is called *double-blind*. The evidence of health outcomes is collected by doctors but analysed by independent statisticians, and all trials (including negative ones) are put on an open database. A company must have two positive trials to go through to the next level and get marketing authorisation. While it's true that doctors sometimes lie about their patients' health outcomes or put the wrong patients in the trial, this really isn't common, and every other aspect of the data is very transparent. These days it's basically impossible to get an ineffective or harmful drug authorised, and in fact, many common medications approved in the past wouldn't be licensed today (including aspirin and paracetamol, because of their toxic effects on the stomach and liver, respectively).

The majority of my own research is publicly funded, but of course I also do research on drugs produced by pharmaceutical companies since many of these are the result of cutting-edge science and so critical to progressing the field on brain research and addiction. Given the transparent nature of data collection and the hoops pharmaceutical companies must jump through to get a drug approved, we're unlikely to end up with ineffective or harmful medication. In fact the greater danger is that pharmaceutical companies stop trying to produce drug treatments for certain conditions altogether, because the approval process is so difficult. This is particularly the case for mental-health disorders, where it is hard to carry out effective trials because of the types of people that have these disorders, and the large number of confounding factors. There is already a strong conservative streak within the pharmaceutical industry, tending to avoid new avenues of research, preferring instead to investigate slight variations on existing drugs that are more likely to reach the marketplace and recoup the development costs. This is understandable given that [†]developing a new medication now costs about $1 billion. However, it leaves lots of promising areas under-researched. If big Pharma stops producing drugs for mental-health disorders altogether and we don't have some alternative way of producing these drugs, it will be immensely damaging to people with mental illness, especially as we are currently in the midst of something of a mental-health epidemic.

The mental-health epidemic

[†]Mental health is the biggest health burden in Europe today, costing more than heart disease and cancer combined. The leading problem for men is alcoholism, and the leading problem for women is depression. There is an urgent need for better treatments and better drugs.

Part of the problem in the UK is that GPs have very little background in mental-health issues – usually about 15 weeks out of their entire training. Yet this is the number-one health problem that they will be diagnosing and attempting to treat in their practice. Of course, GPs have a very high patient load, but the longer a mental-health problem continues without effective treatment, the worse it will get, making the GP even more overworked. Our health service will be vastly improved if much more emphasis is put on dealing with mental-health issues when they first appear, especially because many ill people self-medicate with "recreational" drugs in the absence of prescription medication. These patients often reappear in the medical system many years later with addictions and other health problems from the toxic effects of what they've taken. About a quarter of male alcoholics are thought to have an undiagnosed anxiety disorder, which could probably have been treated successfully with SSRIs if it had been identified before they started drinking heavily. Once they are addicted to alcohol, however, it is much harder to find effective treatments.

Doctors need to have a greater understanding of disorders like depression, and how pharmaceutical and psychological treatments can interact to be most effective – neither is a replacement for the other, and in fact they tend to work best in conjunction. Patients ought to be more involved in their own treatment, weighing up the risks and benefits of the different drugs and treatments available and being allowed to make decisions for themselves. While it's increasingly recognised in the treatment of physical "lifestyle" illnesses (such as obesity and diabetes) that patients should be more active in their own health care, it's *particularly* necessary with mental-health problems because only the patient can know whether the treatment is working. (You can't have a blood test to find out if you're not depressed any more – you have to tell the doctor yourself.)

Of course, from a doctor's point of view it can be difficult to judge when somebody is well enough to make decisions for themselves. Many extremely depressed people, for example, consider committing suicide when they're at their lowest ebb, but once they've received a course of SSRIs feel better and are glad that they weren't allowed to end their lives when they were ill. Or consider force-feeding people with anorexia nervosa. When the body drops below a certain weight, the brain stops working properly and the patient can no longer think rationally. At this point, they can't engage in therapy or decide what other sorts of treatment they might want, so an appropriate treatment is to force-feed them until their brains work again.

This process of stabilising a patient can be very difficult, and needs a lot of trust, especially as many of the drugs prescribed for mental health problems will make patients feel worse initially. It's often difficult to make the correct diagnosis at first, and it's possible that several different courses of drugs will have to be tried before an effective one is found. The expertise of the doctor is crucial at this stage, and a trusting therapeutic relationship is essential. Unfortunately, once a patient has been stabilised many doctors don't want to let the patient have more control over their

Drugs – without the hot air, David Nutt

treatment. This can be very distressing for the patient, and also means the treatment is less likely to work, because treating mental health disorders always requires active engagement of the patient: they won't get better if they're just passively expecting the drugs to do it all for them. Ultimately, the patient is the true expert in their own condition, because they're the one experiencing it.

Informed consent

In recent years, there have been several incidents of effective medications being withdrawn by the pharmaceutical companies themselves (rather than by regulatory bodies) when a small number of patients developed severe side-effects. Of course such side-effects are extremely unfortunate when they do occur; however, for people suffering from very serious illnesses where currently approved medications are considerably less effective than a new drug, or where their medications already carry substantial side-effects, they may think that even very serious complications are worth the possible benefits. Pharmaceutical companies are understandably fearful of litigation, but since it is the patient who will suffer the consequences if something goes wrong it is nonsensical that they can't be allowed to decide to take this risk, especially as we routinely allow much greater levels of risk-taking when people undergo surgery. With invasive procedures, a patient is allowed to face even a very substantial risk of death through informed consent. [†]Up to 1 in 7 elderly patients die after surgery – a level of risk that would never be allowed with a drug.

Rather than allowing regulatory bodies or pharmaceutical companies to decide which drugs are made available to patients, perhaps we could develop a new model for approving drugs based on [†]informed consent. This is a well-established process: the possible dangers of a surgical procedure are explained in layman's terms, and the patient's formal consent protects those who perform the procedure from litigation should there be an adverse outcome. Applying this principle to new drugs would facilitate the current trajectory of medical research, which is increasingly towards "personalised medicine". These are medications tailored to particular genotypes or other specific biological qualities, that will be very beneficial to some people but might be harmful to others. However, because drugs regulation is largely based on risks and benefits averaged across a whole population, positive outcomes for identifiable minorities are often overlooked, and further research on these drugs grinds to a halt, fuelling a risk-averse approach to drug development, which in turn prevents people with serious conditions getting the therapies that could help them. Informed consent could overcome some of this risk-aversion, and would be far more in tune with modern concepts of patient empowerment and shared decision-making than paternalistically removing drugs from the market altogether.

Conclusion

As we discussed in chapter 4, on a day-to-day basis it's considered normal to take drugs to change our brain chemistry – we drink coffee to make us more alert, alcohol to calm us down and take painkillers when we hurt ourselves. Using drugs on prescription for longer-term problems is safer than self-medicating with "recreational" drugs because the former have been through extensive trials to establish safe dosage, and because your doctor can monitor your drug use. The social context of medicinal drug-taking also decreases how pleasurable a drug is, protecting patients from addiction. But prescription drugs do carry some risks, and weighing up the harms against the benefits has to be done on an individual basis – what works for one person may be less beneficial for another, and doctors and patients may have to try multiple treatment options before they find one that is effective. While a doctor's expertise is no less essential than in the past, the medical profession increasingly recognises that the active engagement of patients in their own healthcare is an essential part of getting better. The NHS increasingly emphasises shared decision-making between patients and doctors, but GPs need much more training and support to incorporate this into their practice when encountering mental-health problems.

Drugs – without the hot air, David Nutt

There are many promising avenues for drugs research, and it's possible that we'll be able to turn the tide on the mental-health epidemic as new sorts of treatment are developed. On the scientific side, the field is moving extremely quickly and our knowledge of the brain and of brain disorders expands significantly each year. However, this research cannot solve the problem on its own. It needs funding, from pharmaceutical companies or from the public purse; it needs a political context which allows researchers to explore the potential benefits of drugs even if they're illegal; it needs well-trained medical professionals able to prescribe therapeutic drugs and other forms of treatment appropriately; and it needs a well-informed public who are permitted to make decisions about the best course of treatment for their own mental health.

Notes

Page

217 14% of older people in the UK take them every night• *Drugs and the Future: Brain Science, Addiction and Society*, David Nutt et al, Elsevier, 2007

218 80% of the subjects, who had taken benzodiazepines for an average of 17 years to help them sleep, stopped without any trouble• *Drugs and the Future: Brain Science, Addiction and Society*, David Nutt et al, Elsevier, 2007

221 they have fewer side effects and almost no abuse potential.• *Death and dependence: current controversies over the selective serotonin reuptake inhibitors*, David Nutt, Journal of Psychopharmacology 17(4), December 2003

227 developing a new medication now costs about $1 billion• *Drugs and the Future: Brain Science, Addiction and Society*, David Nutt et al, Elsevier, 2007

227 Mental health is the biggest health burden in Europe today, costing more than heart disease and cancer combined• *Cost of disorders of the brain in Europe 2010*, Gustavsson, A., et al., European Neuropsychopharmacology, 2011

229 Up to 1 in 7 elderly patients die after surgery• *Tens of thousands of surgical patients dying needlessly because of poor NHS care, says Royal College of Surgeons*, Sophie Borland, URL-113, September 29th 2011

229 informed consent.• *Informed consent – a new approach to drug regulation?*, David Nutt, Journal of Psychopharmacology, January 2006

13 Can drugs improve performance?

Over the last two centuries, there has been a great deal of interest in the idea that the new, potently-psychoactive substances we were discovering might be able to increase our physical and mental abilities. Drugs seemed to be able to improve physical performance by keeping us calm under pressure, or building muscle and power, resulting in increased performance and pace. The sports world then began to ban these substances on the grounds that they were unfair and may be physically harmful to athletes. The list of banned drugs has grown ever longer over the past 50 years, even though the evidence linking many of these drugs to improved sporting achievements is rather inconclusive.

Another aspect of performance that drugs can improve is cognition – helping us stay awake, or concentrate, or think more creatively. Stimulants like Ritalin and modafinil are widely used as "study drugs", and in this chapter we look at whether these give users an unfair advantage; we also discuss the most common cognition enhancer: caffeine.

Muscle and power

Using highly potent drugs to improve performance in sport dates back to the early 1800s, when a [†]participant in an "endurance walk" used laudanum to keep himself awake for 24 hours. By the end of the 19th century, [†]nitroglycerin (which is used to stop angina) was commonly used to keep cyclists awake in six-day marathon races. [†]Strychnine was openly used by some long-distance runners, and drugs including cocaine were used both recreationally and for performance by cyclists in the Tour de France. Most of these drugs had the potential for severe side-effects and some athletes came close to death while competing, or suffered from hallucinations and other psychological disturbances.

While amphetamines also were commonly used in the past to increase strength, it's unclear whether these sorts of stimulants really make you any stronger – they might just make you *think* you're doing better, giving you a mental edge. However, they also reduce your control: a famous case was ⁺the death of British cyclist Tommy Simpson. He died on a hill-climb in the Tour de France on a blisteringly hot day, after drinking far too little water, and mixing brandy with two vials of amphetamines. He started cycling erratically, swerving across the road, and eventually collapsed and died. What makes this case particularly tragic is that it's unlikely the drugs helped him cycle any faster. What they *did* do was allow him to ignore the warning signs of overexertion and overheating which would have forced him to stop much earlier, and would probably have saved his life.

GHB has become popular among bodybuilders in recent years, to promote deep sleep after training, because this is when growth hormone is released. Some now inject growth hormone directly.

However, it is drugs called *anabolic steroids* that are most commonly used to build muscle and increase strength. They are taken by thousands of members of the general public, not just professional sports-people. Because anabolic steroids are ⁺the most-widely used performance enhancer, they almost certainly cause the most harm, which is why we focus on them here.

What are anabolic steroids?

⁺Anabolic steroids are synthetic drugs that mimic male sex hormones, particularly testosterone. Their technical name is *anabolic-androgenic steroids*: the *anabolic* part means they stimulate growth, and the *androgenic* part means they "produce maleness". They are used medicinally to stimulate the growth of muscle and bone, for example to treat patients with AIDS wasting syndrome, or to help boys with delayed puberty who aren't producing enough testosterone themselves. They are also used to treat anaemia, and to help male transsexuals in the transition from their original female body (which has more of the sex hormone oestrogen) to their desired male body (which has more testosterone). Finally, there is ongoing research into using them as a male contraceptive.

Researchers have attempted to separate the anabolic and androgenic functions of this type of drug because they're not always desirable at the same time. (For example, when treating women and children, masculine features such as facial hair growth are very undesirable.) However, the two functions have not been dissociated so far.

(Anabolic steroids are sometimes confused with corticosteroids, which are prescribed for conditions like arthritis and asthma and are often referred to simply as "steroids" as well. The difference between the two sorts of steroid is that anabolic steroids increase protein production and hence muscle mass, whereas corticosteroids such as cortisol and prednisolone are anti-stress and anti-inflammatory agents, and cause muscle wasting.)

Who uses anabolic steroids?

Anabolic steroids are usually used by bodybuilders and people who spend a lot of time in the gym or playing sports, as they help build up muscle, and they increase strength by speeding the rate at which people respond to training. As a result, they are banned in most sports, and if a professional is found with them in their bloodstream they will have their medals stripped from them and could be totally banned from the sport for several years.

The British Crime Survey (BCS) estimates that around 50,000 adults use anabolic steroids every year, but this is likely to be a considerable underestimate. The BCS is a door-to-door survey, so it under-represents people who live in group accommodation (such as students and prisoners), those who work in the evenings, and those who spend a lot of their time out of the house, for example at the gym. These are all groups who are more likely to use anabolic steroids. In addition, a secretive sub-culture surrounds the use of anabolic steroids, and many people are unlikely to be honest about whether or not they take them. The proportion of young people who have tried them rose from 0.2% in 2001 to 0.5% in 2006, and if this trend has continued the proportion will be even higher now of course. Most users are primarily interested in increased strength and power, but some take them for aesthetic reasons, attempting to achieve an ideal body type. This group of users is very under-studied, and may have more in common with people with body dysmorphobia (eg anorexia) than with other drug users or athletes.

What are the harms of anabolic steroids?

Anabolic steroids are not known to cause death in overdose, although some long-term users have developed fatal liver problems including cancer, and there have been case reports of people committing suicide on stopping. There have been other cases of users having heart attacks, and suffering acute liver injury. They also lead to damage of tendons and ligaments, as these don't grow as fast as the surrounding muscle. Most users inject, exposing themselves to all the usual risks associated with injection: abscesses, infections and blood-borne viruses such as HIV and hepatitis B and C. Because anabolic steroid users have been far less of a focus in public-health campaigns than other injecting drug users, they may have less knowledge about how to dispose of their used needles safely, which may cause local environmental issues, although their interest in health and in their body makes them less likely to share needles.

Because anabolic steroids are sex hormones, they have quite different effects depending on the age and gender of the person taking them. Their androgenic (male-producing) qualities mean that men are far more likely to use them than women: the ratio of male to female users is about 10 to 1. Women may find their bodies becoming more masculine, growing extra body hair, their voice becoming deeper, their breasts disappearing, and their periods stopping – changes which can be very distressing and may be permanent. On the other hand, men may find their own testosterone production gets suppressed. This is analogous to cocaine causing lower levels of dopamine to be produced naturally by the brain (page 138) – the body recognises that it has enough androgenic hormones coming in from the anabolic steroids and stops producing its own supply. This can lead to sexual dysfunction, the growth of breast tissue, and infertility. These effects can be particularly disruptive if the user has not yet reached full physical maturity, so it's very important that young men are informed of the risks before they consider starting on these drugs.

Case reports have linked the drugs to psychological changes such as mania, depression and increased aggression, though it's possible that users are able to recognise feelings such as aggression and channel them into training or competing harder in their chosen sport. It's hard to know whether anabolic steroids are addictive, but for some people stopping is clearly distressing or difficult. In men, this may be due to the suppression of their own testosterone production – a kind of "testosterone withdrawal" which makes them feel depressed and lethargic without the drugs.

Most people who take anabolic steroids are poly drug users, taking other drugs such as human growth hormone and insulin at the same time. They usually take each steroid in a different way in a practice known as "stacking". For example, they may inject one and take the other orally, in the belief that this will have a greater effect, although this has never been tested. In addition, there is some evidence that many steroid users also take cocaine, and we need more research on the interaction between the two drugs.

How can we reduce the harms of anabolic steroids?

Like benzodiazepines, anabolic steroids are in Class C of the Misuse of Drugs Act, and Schedule 4 of the Medicines Act. This means it is not illegal to buy or possess amounts for personal use, although it is illegal to import with intent to supply. One important but simple harm-reduction measure would be to provide better information about the legal status of the drugs, as many users believe that possession is illegal and therefore don't seek help or treatment.

Another harm reduction measure recommended by the ACMD in their 2010 report would be to make them illegal to import unless they're in someone's possession, and prohibit their sale and purchase online. Buying from the internet can be unsafe as there is very little quality control – products are often contaminated with other substances (which is especially problematic if the drug is going to be injected) and their strength is very variable, making it hard for people to judge dosage.

Other drugs in sport

Drugs are often banned from sports out of fear that they might improve performance and pace, even if there's little evidence that they do. In 2003, American sprinter [†]Kelli White was stripped of her 100 m and 200 m gold medals at the World Championship after a sample tested positive for modafinil, a mild stimulant similar to Ritalin. She claimed that she used it to treat a medical condition, and avoided a two-year ban from the sport after arguing that she didn't think she had to declare it because it wasn't on the list of banned substances at the time. Modafinil was added to this list in January 2004, although it's doubtful that it actually makes people run any faster.

Another question is whether stimulants like amphetamines should be permitted in aerobatics and other activities involving flying. A few years ago, I was contacted by the British Aerobatic Association, who wanted to know if there was any evidence on the effects of stimulants on flying as they were considering a ban on their use. Although this hasn't been formally researched, we do have case studies from the Second World War: [†]the German air force used methamphetamine heavily, which if anything seemed to hinder pilots' abilities in the air. Although stimulants can help people stay awake, they can also get people locked into stereotyped routines, making them less able to respond to the world around them. For that reason I recommended that testing for stimulants was not likely to be worthwhile for aerobatics.

Drugs for calmness in sports

In most sports the concern is that drugs give an unfair advantage because of increased strength or speed. However, in some other sports, such as shooting, the modern pentathlon, winter sports and archery, contestants can improve their performance by taking alcohol or beta blockers to help keep them calm under pressure and prevent muscle tremor (shaking). Most sports now ban these drugs, although alcohol is still permitted in darts even though it may well help keep players' hands steady.

Alcohol is a good example of how the advantage conferred by a drug can be very dose-dependent. At low doses, alcohol can help us keep calm and so improve our accuracy because trembling hands put us at a disadvantage, but at higher doses our coordination deteriorates and our performance declines. If we drink so much that we become dependent on alcohol, however, we can end up with the shakes if we *don't* drink. Any sports person who becomes physically dependent on a drug will find that, although it improves their performance by taking them out of withdrawal, it undermines their ability to perform overall, and they would have been better off if they'd never taken the drug in the first place.

Improving mental performance – cognition enhancers

Cognition enhancers promote certain sorts of brain processing, by improving memory or concentration. Modafinil, a stimulant similar to Ritalin, has started to be used quite widely to maintain vigilance for long periods of time, by people such as soldiers, truck drivers, night-shift workers and students. In World War II, most combatants on both sides were given amphetamines to help them stay awake for long periods when required. Obviously, falling asleep when driving or flying is very dangerous; stimulants can be very useful in these circumstances, though modern health and safety legislation removes the need for this by requiring proper rest periods. Attempts have been made to use stimulants to enhance work performance more widely in society, for example in Russian factories in the Soviet era, but whether there is any net benefit is hard to determine as the need for "catch-up" sleep is always there and these drugs do have adverse effects.

Another set of people who benefit from stimulants, particularly modafinil, are those who don't sleep well at night and suffer from daytime sleepiness.

A debate has begun recently about whether drugs such as modafinil should be banned during exams, or in the study periods leading up to them, as they may confer an unfair advantage. This is quite problematic, not only because this would be very difficult to police, but also because it would raise questions about other common stimulants like nicotine and caffeine. Should they be banned before exams as well? In any case, it has not been proved that modafinil is particularly beneficial to learning. It certainly can allow people to stay awake and work for longer before they need to sleep, so increasing the total time available for study. But whether this translates into improved exam performance is not known. Different sorts of cognitive tasks require different sorts of brain processing, and sometimes taking drugs to improve one type of thinking makes it more difficult to engage in another. In clinical practice, some patients on Ritalin and other stimulants say that the drug reduces their mental flexibility, so they feel over-focused, less creative, and engage in fewer tasks.

Which aspects of cognition you want to enhance depends a lot on the circumstances and what you're trying to achieve. One alternative "cognition enhancer" is the cannabis smoked by many musicians, who say it improves their creativity and appreciation of music even if it also impairs other processes such as memory formation. Heavy use of psychedelics can have a negative effect on some cognitive processes, but can also reveal new ways of thinking, inspiring not just writers like Aldous Huxley but scientists like Nobel prizewinner Kary Mullis (see next chapter). In the future, we may find ways to isolate the positive benefits that drugs can bring to the way we think, while minimising the downsides.

Is my child addicted to Ritalin?

In recent years, prescribing stimulants to people with ADHD (attention deficit hyperactivity disorder), has been controversial. The drug most commonly used for this is methylphenidate, a mild form of amphetamine (sold under the names Ritalin or Concerta). There are several aspects to the controversy. Some people deny that ADHD really exists, or think it is a real disorder but that stimulants are an inappropriate way to treat it. Others think that, even if *some* people really do have ADHD and benefit from Ritalin, the drug is being prescribed inappropriately in a very large proportion of cases, particularly for children whose parents may just be finding their normal childish energy challenging.

Case study

I met a 15-year-old girl who had had terrible behavioural problems from about the age of 9 until she was 14. She had been removed from mainstream schooling and her parents had had to drive for several hours each day to the special school she was placed in. Her parents were insistent that she had ADHD but for years the professionals involved in her care refused to consider Ritalin because they didn't accept the diagnosis. Eventually, after battling long and hard, she was given a dose of Ritalin; within about half an hour she was able to sit still and calm, and had a proper conversation with her mother for the first time in years. She then went back into mainstream education and passed her GCSEs whilst receiving this treatment. However, when she left home she came under a new doctor who did not believe in the diagnosis or treatment, and stopping her medication. She immediately relapsed and dropped out of further education. When I saw her later, her condition had deteriorated to the point where restarting the medication was not able to restore her function, so her prospects of a normal life were ruined.

ADHD is a disorder characterised by a range of symptoms including a very short attention span, an inability to concentrate or sit still even if the surroundings are peaceful and calm, impulsive behaviour such as acting without thinking, and having little or no sense of danger. Children with the disorder may also have other problems such as dyslexia, but even if they don't, they are likely to under-perform in school because they can't focus on the tasks that they've been set. The result for many children is that they lose confidence in their abilities and stop trying, which can cause huge problems throughout the rest of their lives. We can often recognise a child with ADHD because they seem to be under-performing compared with what their IQ would suggest they are capable of. ADHD is often treated with Ritalin. Ritalin is a dopamine reuptake inhibitor, which blocks dopamine transporters in the brain in a similar way to cocaine. However, when taken orally it takes about an hour for concentrations in the brain to peak (compared with about five minutes for cocaine). So although when it arrives it works very efficiently –[†]blocking around 50% of dopamine transporters – it doesn't produce a "high" and is unlikely to cause addiction. It's only when Ritalin is taken in non-prescribed ways – for example when it's injected or when crushed up pills are snorted – that it reaches the brain much faster, and this is when addiction can occur.

A child who needs Ritalin to function normally is not addicted. If they had diabetes they would need insulin every day and would suffer physical problems without it, but we wouldn't consider them "addicted" to insulin. Many young people who take these sort of stimulants don't really like them – they're not pleasurable, they can cause headaches and nausea, and make the person feel "too focused" and not spontaneous. As a result young people often stop of their own accord when they reach adolescence (even though this may worsen their educational performance, because many people do find they benefit significantly from the drug long into adulthood).

Addiction *can* occur where Ritalin is diverted: people who have it on prescription either take too much in one go, or sell it to others who don't have prescriptions. Intravenous use is rare. Snorting is more common, making the drug both more addictive and more harmful than when taken orally. Snorting any drug can damage the nose, and injecting carries the dangers of blood-borne viruses, abscesses and skin problems. In the USA, so many children are taking psychoactive prescription medication that there is a lot of diversion of Ritalin and other drugs amongst school children. While there isn't much evidence of this happening in the UK at present, it is certainly a risk that needs to be taken into account.

Although the rapid rise in the number of people being diagnosed with ADHD and prescribed stimulants has led to fears of "over-medication", [†]we still estimate that only about a quarter of those who would benefit from them are currently taking them. Indeed, the opposite – not prescribing them because of doubts about the disorder – seems to be as much of a problem as excessive keenness to medicate. (However, there may indeed be cases where Ritalin is misused; we doctors don't always try non-medical treatments when they would be appropriate.)

Young people with ADHD are often very good at some specfic activities such as playing video games, and it may well be that experimenting with different teaching techniques, and computer games to train the brain, would be just as beneficial as drugs. But for now, prescribing stimulants for ADHD sufferers at least gives them a chance to succeed in our current school system.

The most common cognition enhancer: coffee

[†]Coffee originates from East Africa (where it grows in the same sort of terrain as khat). There are different stories about how and when humans first started to consume coffee, some of which suggest we copied birds and goats who seemed to enjoy the stimulating properties of the berries. The raw berries are bitter and unpleasant to humans, however, and it takes quite a lot of technical expertise to turn them into a palatable drink. It's difficult to know if these techniques were actually learnt around the 8th or 9th centuries, as the myths suggest, or if they only developed shortly before the first written accounts of coffee drinking, in Yemen in the mid-15th century.

As coffee spread throughout the Muslim world and on to Europe, it was met with concern at first. Attempts were made to ban it as unIslamic or unChristian, but its popularity made these bans ineffective, and soon huge numbers of coffee houses had sprung up – over [†]3000 in England alone by 1675. Having been criticised for causing illness, coffee now began to be credited with the ability to cure all sorts of ailments, from stomach problems to headaches. It is now the most-commonly used drug in the world, and it's taste is so popular we now even have a non-active version – decaffeinated coffee.

How does coffee work?

The active ingredient in coffee is caffeine, which is also present in tea and chocolate (though in smaller quantities). When the brain engages in metabolic activity, it produces a small molecule called adenosine as a byproduct, which builds up in the brain and makes you feel tired – a bit like mental lactic acid. Caffeine blocks the effects of adenosine, which is why it makes you feel more awake (and why [†]your sensitivity to caffeine depends partly on what sort of adenosine receptors you have.)

Historically, there was much concern about caffeine addiction when coffee was first introduced; for example, Bach wrote a cantata about a woman whose father wanted her to give up her coffee habit. This kind of concern was very common, but in fact even heavy users are rarely actually addicted in the true sense: they don't experience cravings when they stop, or suffer distress if they have to go without. In contrast, most people *are* physically dependent on caffeine without their knowledge: they will go into withdrawal if they don't have it. This causes the familiar Saturday morning headache of those who routinely drink lots of strong coffee at work and then stop at the week end. So, while coffee drinkers are usually physically dependent, they are not addicted.

Does coffee improve performance?

It's difficult to be sure whether coffee actually improves performance. Most of us are physically dependent on it, going into withdrawal overnight, and withdrawal impairs performance. If a coffee drinker does better on a task after having some caffeine it's difficult to know whether this is a genuine improvement or just compensating for the impairment they experienced before they had their caffeine fix (ie not a positive factor, just the removal of a negative factor). This theory is supported by research which has found that [†]caffeine improves performance more in people who are coffee drinkers than those who normally don't consume caffeine at all. On the other hand, caffeine certainly does have effects in itself – researchers use it to model insomnia when they're testing sleeping pills, for example – so it's possible it does provide a mild cognitive advantage.

Conclusion

When new drugs first appear, they're often hailed as "wonder drugs" – able to overcome human limitations of fear, tiredness and depression. When Sigmund Freud first tried cocaine, for example, he described the experience as one of:

> †*"exhilaration and lasting euphoria, which in no way differs from the normal euphoria of the healthy person ... You perceive an increase of self-control and possess more vitality and capacity for work ...Long intensive mental or physical work is performed without any fatigue ... Absolutely no craving for the further use of cocaine appears after the first, or even after repeated taking of the drug."*

Of course it didn't take long for people to work out that, not only is cocaine highly addictive after all, but that no drug can actually give you more energy – it can delay fatigue, but you'll have to come down at some point, and the longer you put it off, the harder you will crash on the other side. So it's debatable whether drugs really do help people to improve their physical performance, as the side-effects of many drugs soon start to outweigh their benefits. This applies to mental tasks as well. A drug that helps you stay awake may lock you into stereotypical routines, and a drug that allows you to concentrate for really long periods may make it harder for you to think creatively.

The quest for improved mental and physical performance poses ethical issues about the sorts of drugs that we want to develop and the sorts of purposes we want them for. In chapter 16 we'll be looking at the future of drugs – where drug research is taking us, and the sorts of decisions that might face us in the years to come.

Notes

Page

232 participant in an "endurance walk" used laudanum to keep himself awake for 24 hours• *Dopage: l'imposture des performances*, Jean Pierre de Mondernard, Willmett II Chiron, 2000

232 nitroglycerin (which is used to stop angina) was commonly used to keep cyclists awake in six-day marathon races• *Use of performance-enhancing drugs in sport*, Wikipedia, URL-32.

232 Strychnine was openly used by some long-distance runners• *La Fabuleuse Histoire des Jeux Olympiques*, Robert Pariente and Guy Lagorce, Minerva, 2004

233 the death of British cyclist Tommy Simpson• *British riders remember Tommy Simpson – a hero to some, to others the villain of the Ventoux*, URL-114, Richard Moore, July 26th 2009

233 the most-widely used performance enhancer• *Conveniently, they are also the most-widely studied.*

233 Anabolic steroids are synthetic drugs• *Consideration of the Anabolic Steroids*, ACMD, URL-115, September 2010

237 Kelli White was stripped of her 100 m and 200 m gold medals• *Sprinter likely to lose medals*, New York Times, URL-116, September 10th 2003

237 the German air force used methamphetamine heavily• *Concepts of Chemical Dependency*, Harold E. Doweiko, Cengage Learning, 2009

241 blocking around 50% of dopamine transporters• *Methylphenidate and cocaine have a similar in vivo potency to block dopamine transporters in the human brain*, Nora Volkow et al, Life Sciences 65 (1), May 28th 1999

241 we still estimate that only about a quarter of those who would benefit from them are currently taking them• *Service contacts among the children participating in the British Child and Adolescent Mental Health Surveys*, T Ford, H Hamilton and R Goodman, Child and Adolescent Mental Health 10, 2005. The authors examine the most severe form of ADHD: hyperkinetic disorder.

242 Coffee originates from East Africa (where it grows in the same sort of terrain as khat)• *Exotic Substances: the introduction and global spread of tobacco, coffee, cocoa, tea and distilled liquor, sixteenth to eighteenth centuries*, Rudi Matthee, in Drugs and Narcotics in History, Cambridge University Press, 1995

242 3000 in England alone by 1675• *Wake up and smell the coffee in Turkey's beautiful Izmir*, author, URL-119, August 25th 2011

243 your sensitivity to caffeine depends partly on what sort of adenosine receptors you have.• *Association of the anxiogenic and alerting effects of caffeine with ADORA2A and ADORA1 polymorphisms and habitual level of caffeine consumption.* PJ Rogers, C Hohoff, SV Heatherley, EL Mullings, PJ Maxfield, RP Evershed, J Deckert and DJ Nutt, Neuropsychopharmacology 35: 1973–83, 2010

243 caffeine improves performance more in people who are coffee drinkers than those who normally don't consume caffeine at all• *Association of the anxiogenic and alerting effects of caffeine with ADORA2A polymorphisms and habitual level of caffeine consumption*, Peter Rogers et al, Neuropsychopharmacology, 35, 2010

244 "exhilaration and lasting euphoria, which in no way differs from the normal euphoria of the healthy person ... • *Uber Coca*, Sigmund Freud, *Centralblatt für die gestalt Therapie*, 1884

14 Psychedelics – should scientists try LSD?

Psychedelic drugs have been used by humans for millennia, probably longer than any other sort of drug because they occur in edible fungi. (The Avenue des Champs Elysees in Paris is named after the Elysian Fields in ancient Greece, where people went annually to eat psychedelic mushrooms and experience "trips".) However, psychedelics remain the least understood drugs in neuroscience. The word "psychedelic" comes from the Greek for "mind-manifesting", referring to one of these drugs' most remarkable qualities – that they reveal the inner workings of people's minds. LSD, a synthetic compound that was discovered by accident, is the best-known and most-studied psychedelic, and its story also shows how the cultural context of a drug's emergence can affect how it is classified and controlled. Other psychedelics that we will discuss briefly include magic mushrooms, ayuesca, peyote and ibogaine.

How do psychedelics work?

All psychedelics directly stimulate a particular subtype of our serotonin receptors; these are the 5HT2A receptors and play an important role in higher, cortical, brain functions. The best-known effect is the production of unusual visuals – not true hallucinations (which are images that have no basis in reality), but strange distortions and imaginative additions to images of the things that are physically present. These can happen both with eyes open and eyes closed. Psychedelic drugs are also *empathogenic* – they create sensations of care, love, and connection to other people and to the natural world. It's still a mystery why these natural products and their derivatives produce visual effects, whereas synthetic SSRIs (which also increase levels of serotonin) just produce changes in mood and energy. It's unlikely we'll be able to unravel this mystery fully as long as psychedelics remain illegal and research on them is so restricted.

Modern brain-imaging techniques have shown us that the brain works in many different modes: acting, seeing, listening, planning and attention, moving, feeling, etc. One is called the "default mode", which includes normal "housekeeping" functions, such as memory, self-reflective thought, and the sense of our body in space. Psilocybin, a prototypical psychedelic, switches off this mode [†](Figure 14.1), so disrupting the sense of "self". It seems likely that all psychedelics do the same. People often describe a psychedelic experience as like "seeing the world anew", probably because they break out of the normal routine of brain processing. It's because of this effect that our expert panel rated LSD highest in terms of the drug-specific impairment of mental functioning.

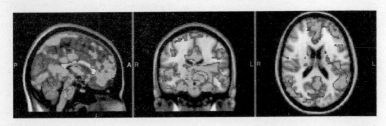

Figure 14.1: Brain scan showing the decreases in blood flow produced by psilocybin. The regions where it reduces brain blood flow are those that make up the default mode network.

The discovery of LSD

For centuries, it was known that a fungus called ergot had peculiar properties. Some of these were purely medicinal. Ergot constricts blood vessels, so extracts were used by midwives to prevent women dying from excessive bleeding after childbirth. This property also helps with migraine headaches, so by the early 1900s purified ergotamine was being used to treat migraine. Other properties were more mysterious. Periodic outbreaks of madness and strange visions amongst whole populations often coincided with particular climatic conditions that caused the fungus to grow on crops of rye. There is [†]a theory that the stories of magic and devils reported by the girls of Salem during their witchcraft trials in 1692 were the result of ergot poisoning.

In the 1930s, a brilliant Swiss chemist called Albert Hofmann, who was working for the pharmaceutical company Sandoz, began studying ergotamines. Most of these ergot-based substances are based on lysergic acid, and Hofmann began combining lysergic acid with other compounds to make new drugs such as dihydroergotamine for migraines, hydergin for circulatory disorders, and methergine for bleeding after childbirth. By 1938 he had created 24 of these new drugs based on ergotamine, and he began working on the 25th in the series, combining lysergic acid with a compound based on nicotinic acid diethylamide, used in medicine to stimulate circulation. The result was lysergic acid diethylamide (LSD), which he produced in November 1938. Pharmacological testing showed this new chemical had no properties of interest, so the company stopped investigating it. But Hofmann had a hunch that something had been missed, and five years later he synthesised another batch.

In the process of making the sample, Hofmann spilt a little of the compound on his fingers. He records that he:

> [†]*"was seized by a peculiar sensation of vertigo and restlessness ... In a dreamlike state, I left for home ... With my eyes closed, fantastic pictures of extraordinary plasticity and intensive colour seemed to surge towards me."*

Realising afterwards that this had probably been caused by exposure to LSD, he decided to take a small amount deliberately – just a quarter of a milligram – to see if it really had been responsible.

It soon became clear that even that tiny dose was considerably stronger than his previous experience. He cycled home with his laboratory assistant, and the sensations became extremely frightening. Later he wrote:

> [†]*"I lost all control of time: space and time became more and more disorganised and I was overcome with fears that I was going crazy ... Occasionally I felt as being outside my body. I thought I had*

> died. My 'ego' was suspended somewhere in space and I saw my
> body lying dead on the sofa."

After about six hours the sensations became less intense, and he woke up the next morning with a great sense of well-being, having had the world's first deliberate LSD trip.

LSD and psychiatry

The discovery of the psychedelic properties of LSD coincided with several other breakthroughs in neuroscience that completely revolutionised our understanding of the brain and mental illness. Until then, the principal framework for understanding mental illness was the one provided by psychoanalysis: people went mad because of repressed traumatic experiences which needed to be exposed through the "talking cure" pioneered by Freud. Although this approach had undoubtedly been beneficial to many people, it had been largely ineffective for those with more severe disorders such as schizophrenia.

The discovery that LSD could create symptoms similar to psychosis coincided with the identification of serotonin and its presence in the brain. Together, these discoveries helped develop a new understanding, based on brain chemistry, of psychotic disturbances. This is one of the reasons why drug-control laws that limit research on psychoactive substances are so damaging to neuroscience: so much of what we know about brain chemistry, neurotransmitters, receptors, and how to treat the most severe types of mental illness, has been learned from studying the changes induced by (now-illegal) drugs that change the way we see the world.

Hofmann immediately recognised that his new compound could be beneficial to psychiatry. The first thing he did was inform several of his pharmacologist colleagues, who repeated his experiment with similar results. The drug was then taken by a group of psychiatrists in Canada, including Humphrey Osmond, Abram Hoffer and Duncan Blewett, all working at the Saskatchewan hospital in North Battleford. An immediate result was they changed how they personally approached their patients – [†]they recorded that they found themselves taking their schizophrenic patients' accounts of their illness more seriously after being put in their shoes for a while. They then began doing experiments on patients, paying great attention to the "set" and "setting" of the experience.

Set and setting

More than any other sort of drug, psychedelics show the importance of "set" and "setting" in creating a drug experience. The *set* is what you bring to it – your own background and state of mind, previous encounters with changing your brain chemistry, and expectations of what's going to happen. The *setting* is the environment where you consume the drug – whether it's known and familiar, who you're with and how they're behaving, whether you're indoors or outside, the music, the light. We all know that drinking a bottle of wine quietly at home will have quite different effects to drinking the same amount in a noisy pub; with psychedelics, the difference between a positive and negative set and setting can be the difference between life-changing insights into your own psychology, and a deeply-disturbing psychosis-like experience.

†The LSD trials at Saskatchewan were held in a loving and calm environment. A guide was present to reassure the drug taker if they felt afraid, but who was otherwise "self-effacing" – not imposing themselves on the experience. People were screened psychologically before they were accepted onto the trials, and given a lot of preparation about what was likely to happen. Afterwards, they could join support groups to discuss what had happened, with others who'd been through the same thing. The circumstances were conducive to a positive and insightful experience that helped people understand in a new way their own actions and motivations.

Other experiments, however, were less successful. At another mental hospital in Canada staff administered the drug and then tied the patients down to the bed while they were intoxicated. Understandably, their experiences were far less positive. At the same time, the USA military began experimenting with using LSD as a weapon to see if they could immobilise whole populations. Recently-uncovered CIA files suggest that an †outbreak of insanity in the French town of Pont-Saint-Esprit in 1951 may have been the result of American agents deliberately contaminating a batch of bread with the psychedelic, rather than accidental ergot poisoning as was thought at the time. Whatever the cause, since those affected had no expectations about what was going to happen, they were very disturbed by what they experienced.

LSD leaves the laboratory

Hofmann saw his creation as a tool for therapy and spiritual awakening. The quasi-religious uses of the drug were confirmed when analysis of the active ingredients in naturally-occurring psychedelics were found to be very similar to LSD. Magic mushrooms, ayuesca and peyote had all been used for thousands of years by natives of the Americas in religious rituals, and were essential to their cultural understandings of the world. But inevitably, these substances began to draw the attention of people who wanted to use them outside of traditional rituals or the laboratory setting. The most infamous of these was Harvard professor Timothy Leary.

In 1959 †Leary first tried psilocybin, the active ingredient in magic mushrooms, and he soon began experimenting with LSD as well. As someone deeply frustrated by the nature of American society, he thought LSD was the silver bullet that would transform the culture he lived in, from a materialist, self-centred, warlike society to one based on principles of freedom, peace and love. Leary began conducting experiments with both psilocybin and LSD on students and fellow lecturers. At first the university authorities approved of the work, until they realised that Leary had vastly overstepped the remit of the study design he'd agreed to. He and his colleague Richard Alpert were expelled from the university. They then continued their experiments in a mansion they bought in New York State.

Leary was extremely outspoken about his intentions for LSD, which became known colloquially as "acid". He thought that everybody in America should be given it to open their minds to new ways of thinking – they should "turn on, tune in and drop out". Many people tried it and did have positive experiences, but others who weren't warned of the dangers of the wrong set or setting had frightening "bad trips" which made them extremely anxious and distressed. As the downsides of both "good" and "bad" psychedelic experiences became known, LSD began to be seen as highly dangerous, especially as some of those who had had their perspectives changed by the drug started to become politically active.

It's no coincidence that, while LSD was displacing psychoanalysis as the paradigm for understanding the brain in psychiatry, it also displaced the psychoanalytic model of neurosis and "maladjustment". Pyschoanalysis placed all the onus on the individual to conform to the society they lived in rather than trying to change that society so that it was more accepting of a diversity of views and ways of living. Rather than just accepting racism, sexism and homophobia, some people who took LSD started questioning whether these were good cultural values to hold.

Of course, LSD wasn't solely responsible for all the different cultural shifts happening in the 1960s, but it was the archetypal drug of "flower power" and as such became the focus of concern for social conservatives who wanted to preserve the status quo. Conservatives blamed LSD for promoting many different activist movements, from civil-rights protestors and feminists and ecologists, to those opposing the wars in Korea and Vietnam. LSD has been described as the "spiritual antidote to the atom bomb", and even in the experiments carried out by the CIA its peaceful qualities came through. Although the military wanted to use LSD as a weapon of war, many of the soldiers they gave it to responded to the experience by saying they no longer believed in violence and that they wanted to leave the army.

There was a huge backlash, and in 1966 LSD was made a Class A drug in the USA. The UK soon followed suit. Even worse, it was placed in Schedule 1, as having no recognised therapeutic uses, despite warnings from the scientific community that this would seriously harm research into a set of drugs with unique properties for treating mental illness. Leary popularised the drug so that everyone could obtain it on the street, but also led to its prohibition so that it could no longer be used in legitimate research.

What are the harms of LSD and psychedelics?

Although a bad LSD trip can be extremely frightening and distressing, psychedelics overall are among the safest drugs we know of. When the ISCD expert panel were rating LSD and mushrooms (which contain psilocybin) by our 16 criteria, they both scored either 0 or 1 in everything apart from specific and related impairment of mental functioning. It's virtually impossible to die from an overdose of them; they cause no physical harm; and if anything they are anti-addictive, as they cause a sudden tolerance which means that if you immediately take another dose it will probably have very little effect, so there is no incentive to take more.

Psychedelics are unpredictable, and taking them requires the right circumstances and proper psychological preparation – if you took them unknowingly you'd think you were going mad. People with existing mental-health problems such as schizophrenia can find that psychedelics worsen their symptoms, and should probably avoid them unless under medical supervision. In the early days, it was thought that the effects of LSD were a model for schizophrenia, and it's certainly true that taking LSD gives healthy people an insight into that kind of mental disturbance. However, although there is a similar sort of sense of ego fragmentation, psychedelic drugs produce mostly visual changes, while with schizophrenia the hallucinations are mostly auditory (eg [†]"hearing voices"). Psychedelics should probably also be avoided by those who have high levels of anxiety as they'll find the lack of control unsettling. Such people are unlikely to be tempted to take them anyway – some of my patients are so anxious they are frightened to take even an alcoholic drink (let alone take LSD) in case it undermines their sense of self-control.

Obviously there is a greater chance of having an accident if a lot of the normal "housekeeping" functions in the brain aren't operating, although the risk of this is often overstated. For example, there is a common misconception that people who take LSD will start believing they can fly and jump out of windows. There is no evidence that this has ever happened, and it's possible that this apocryphal tale stems from [†]an edition of Spiderman in 1971 where a young man takes LSD and hurls himself off a building, only to be saved by the superhero. (It's worth pointing out that each year dozens of people in the UK severely injure or kill themselves falling out of windows or off balconies and roofs while drunk.)

Undertaking normal activities like driving is a very bad idea if you've taken LSD. Many years ago in the USA, I met a couple of 20-year olds who told me a story about the effects of a recent LSD trip of theirs. They had started driving from New York to New Jersey. They were aware that they were still high from earlier and that they needed to take care on the road. Before very long the police pulled them over, and when they objected that they'd been driving carefully the policeman pointed out they'd been moving at two miles an hour! This occurred because the drug changes the perception of speed as well as time; on Hofmann's first experiment he records feeling that he was hardly moving on his bicycle trip home, although his assistant told him afterwards they'd been going at a normal pace.

What are the benefits of psychedelics?

Not only are psychedelics anti-addictive in themselves, but they may be useful in treating addiction to other drugs. Some of the early trials in Saskatchewan gave LSD to alcoholics, initially with the idea that if it gave them a bad experience it might shock them out of their behaviour. What happened instead was that the psychedelic gave some of them a new perspective on their lives, helping them face up to the damage they were doing to their families and friends, and this new empathy motivated them to change their behaviour. Similar changes in thinking are often reported by alcoholics successfully completing the 12-step AA programme. Since then there have been at least †five other studies that have found LSD helps people overcome alcoholism.

Many people describe psychedelic experiences as profoundly meaningful, which may help them develop a sense of purpose in life or envisage an alternative to being stuck in a rut with alcohol. This may also extend to treating low moods more generally, as many depressed people are stuck in a vicious cycle where their depression prevents them doing anything to alleviate their depression. LSD, psilocybin and similar drugs might open up a different way of thinking, allowing people to improve their situation. (I am now conducting a study funded by the Medical Research Council, to see if we can use a single treatment with psilocybin to help people recover from depression. We expect to have the results around 2015.)

The meaningful experiences induced by LSD and other psychedelics can help people deal with other major problems, such as facing their own death. Experiments with terminal patients have shown that many become much less scared after a psychedelic experience, often because while they're on the drug they've felt as though they've become part of the universe and that some part of them will continue after death. What's remarkable is that usually just a single dose or two can have profound and lasting effects, without creating cravings to repeat the experience. People tend to remember their trips in vivid detail, and keep the insights they've gained for a long time rather than needing to use the drug repeatedly to recreate them.

On the more physiological side, many people who suffer from

[†]cluster headaches self-medicate with psychedelics, which seem to be the only effective therapy for this disorder. These headaches are so severe that they can drive people to the point of suicide. The vasoconstrictive properties (constricting blood vessels in the head) of LSD and magic mushrooms somehow interrupt this pain like no other drugs. As with MS sufferers denied cannabis, and terminal cancer patients denied morphine, it's utterly inhumane that the legal restrictions on these drugs mean that the only way people suffering from these disorders can get the medicine they need is by becoming criminals.

Should scientists take LSD?

One line of enquiry which was being studied before LSD was made illegal was its [†]use in problem solving. This may seem surprising because most people find it hard to focus when tripping, and it's certainly true that people taking LSD don't perform particularly well on standard psychological tests. As psychologist Arthur Kleps explained in 1966, *"if I were to give you an IQ test and during the administration one of the walls of the room opened up giving you a vision of the blazing glories of the central galactic suns, and at the same time your childhood began to unreel before your inner eye like a three-dimensional colour movie, you would not do well on the test."* However, psychedelics can induce creativity, by lowering the psychological defences around "getting something wrong" and helping to see problems from new angles. With the right set and setting, this can be directed towards familiar problems, sometimes with spectacular results.

This approach seems to work best when the problem is one that has been considered many times while sober, and the setting includes notes, lots of paper and pens to record your thoughts, and a guide to help you through the initial disorientation and remind you of what your aim is. Although most people who have tried psychedelics might find it hard to believe that it would be possible to concentrate on a task during a trip, that's probably because they've taken them in circumstances where they were easily distracted – and they've probably also been surrounded by other people on drugs at the same time. In a calm setting it's much easier to focus, and in fact people on LSD are so suggestible that if they have a guide who tells them that they will have no difficulty concentrating, this will probably be the case.

Taking LSD in this way has been known to deliver moments of inspiration to designers, architects and engineers. There are many stories about near-perfect technical designs which have suddenly become obvious while contemplating the problem on the drug. In *LSD – the Problem Solving Psychedelic*, written in 1967, the authors recount several examples of this. One was a furniture designer who completed a chair design while on LSD which was successfully modelled into a functional dining chair with no substantial changes from the original concept. (These pieces of furniture are extremely difficult to create and the designer was used to new chairs taking two months and ten trial models to complete.) Another example was an engineer who worked in Naval Research and had been trying to design an special detection device for five years without success. Within minutes of contemplating the problem on LSD he had found the solution and the device was then patented and used by the US Navy. A third example was an architect who took the drug to help him design a shopping centre and was able to visualise it in its entirety: *"Suddenly I saw the finished project. I did some quick calculations . . . it would fit on the property and not only that . . . it would meet the cost and income requirements . . . I began to draw . . . my senses could not keep up with my images."* The image stayed with him just as sharply after the drug experience had ended, and his design was accepted and constructed.

Even in the less-obviously creative fields of hard science, LSD can be profoundly beneficial. In fact, it played a role in the two biggest discoveries in biology of the 20th century. [†]Francis Crick, who discovered the double helix structure of DNA with James Watson, and [†]Kary Mullis, who invented the [†]polymerase chain reaction (PCR), had both taken the drug, and attributed some of their understanding and insights to it. Mullis has gone so far as to say: *"would I have invented PCR if I hadn't taken LSD? I seriously doubt it . . . [having taken LSD] I could sit on a DNA molecule and watch the polymers go by. I learnt that partly on psychedelic drugs."*

Both Crick and Mullis received Nobel prizes for their work. Now that LSD is illegal few scientists would dare to use it, and even fewer would own up to taking it. Perhaps scientific progress in many areas has been hindered by this state of affairs!

Mushrooms and other psychedelics

[†]There are many other kinds of psychedelic drugs that have different effects to LSD but broadly share the same risks and benefits. The most common ones you're likely to encounter are covered here.

Psilocybin is found in psychedelic "magic" mushrooms. It's inert itself, but breaks down in the body to psilocin, which is a potent pyschoactive substance. Psilocybin is found in mushrooms all over the world: we know most about their history in religious ceremonies in South and Central America, but the Sami in Siberia have a long history of using fly agaric mushrooms in shamanic rituals, and it seems likely that magic

Drugs – without the hot air, David Nutt

mushrooms were used by the ancient Greeks in the Elysian fields. Psilocybin's effects are very similar to LSD, but psilocybin is much shorter-acting, lasting 20 to 30 minutes, so it's much more practical than LSD for use in brain imaging when we study the effects of psychedelics.

DMT (dimethyltriptamine) is the psychoactive ingredient in several species of plants native to South America. There are different traditional methods of consuming these plants, such as shooting *anadenanthera peregrina* out of a pipe into someone's eye, or drinking "ayuesca tea" as part of an elaborate ceremony. Pure DMT can be inhaled (when it lasts 5 to 15 minutes), snorted or injected (when it lasts longer), or taken orally (when it lasts about three hours). When taken orally it has to be combined with a monoamine oxidase inhibitor (MAOI) or it will be broken down too quickly to be effective. Traditional ayuesca tea is made from a mixture of leaves that combine DMT and MAOI; for example, the *psychotria viridis* shrub provides the DMT, and the *banisteriopsis caapi* vine is the source of MAOI. DMT is a Class A drug in the UK, but natural products containing it are not classified.

Mescaline is the psychoactive substance in the peyote cactus, which has been used by for at least 5,000 years by indigenous peoples in present-day Northern Mexico, and the states of Oklahoma and Texas. The fruit of the cactus is dried and boiled into tea. This usually causes extreme nausea before producing psychedelic visuals and states of introspection and insight, which last about 10–12 hours. In 1954, Aldous Huxley was inspired to write *The Doors of Perception* after a mescaline trip; the book played a pivotal role in popularising psychedelics in the 1960s. Although both peyote and mescaline are illegal in the USA, the Native American Church won the right to use the cactus in "bona fide religious ceremonies" in 1996. In the UK, mescaline is a Class A drug.

Ibogaine is the active ingredient in plants of the iboga family, native to West Africa. It's used within medical and ritual ceremonies in the Bwiti cult, primarily in Gabon and Cameroon. It's one of the most long-lasting psychedelics, with trips sometimes going on for days. Ibogaine seems to be able to prevent or minimise withdrawal symptoms from opiates and alcohol, which, combined with the new perspective it gives people on their behaviour, may make it a highly effective treatment for addiction. Several centres around the world are now using this approach, although adequate clinical trials have yet to be conducted so we don't know how safe or effective it is, and it can't be recommended. Ibogaine is legal in the UK.

Why were magic mushrooms banned in the UK?

Psilocybin occurs naturally in over 200 species of fungi which grow in the wild in many parts of the world, including the UK. The species which is native to Britain is *psilocybe semilanceata*, known as "liberty caps", which grow in shady and woodland areas in the autumn. It's unclear how long they've been deliberately used for their psychoactive effects: in the [†]few recorded incidents of people taking them accidentally, the unexpected sensory distortions were experienced as poisoning. Although there are some theories that they were used in pagan rituals in Britain in the past, there's very little evidence of this, and it's possible that their effects were unknown or unappreciated until the 1960s.

Magic mushrooms first came to widespread attention in the west in 1957 after an amateur mycologist and his wife took part in a [†]Valeda mushroom ceremony in Mexico. They recorded their experience in a magazine article, which prompted scientists to start cultivating and investigating different species, and of course Timothy Leary also helped popularise magic mushrooms among hippies. British people picking and eating liberty caps in the autumn, and having largely enjoyable and safe psychedelic experiences in the countryside, was a common, popular and legal pastime until 2005.

In the early 2000s, the British government started to become concerned about magic mushrooms. Some companies had started importing them freeze-dried from the Netherlands and selling them in shops in the Camden area of London, and this was generating bad press in the tabloids. Rather than simply banning their sale, the government decided to act "tough on drugs" and ban their possession altogether. They made a rushed decision to place them in Class A, even though they were clearly much less harmful than other Class A drugs like crack and heroin. (The government argument for categorising them this way was that pure psilocybin was Class A, so the source of the chemical should be as well – although there was little justification for psilocybin being in this Class in the first place.) If they had consulted with us on the ACMD we could have told them that this classification was inappropriate, but in their hurry to be seen to take action they produced a badly-thought-out piece of legislation without seeking our advice at all. (Arguably this was illegal, since consulting with the ACMD is required by law). This was the beginning of the Labour government starting to ignore the ACMD when passing drugs legislation – and the beginning of the end for me.

We now have the ridiculous situation that if you find magic mushrooms in the wild you can sit in the field and munch them to your heart's content, but if you take them home you could go to prison for up to seven years, and if you give them to a friend you'll be supplying a Class A drug and you could spend 14 years in jail. This silliness weakens respect for the law, and makes people distrust the classification system as an objective indicator of the relative harm of different drugs.

Conclusion

The story of LSD and other psychedelics show how the cultural context of a drug can affect our assessment of how dangerous it is. Although psychedelics are among the least harmful psychoactive substances, especially when taken with the right set and setting, they've developed a reputation as things to be feared, and LSD is among the few drugs where there has been a marked decline in use over the last 30 years. In many ways this is a good thing, as bad trips can be extremely unpleasant. However, these sorts of drugs may also be among the most beneficial in the world for treating addiction, depression and other sorts of mental illness, and for advancing science and the arts. In the last few years, LSD trials have begun again in Switzerland, the USA and the UK. Hopefully as the medicinal uses of psychedelics become officially recognised, it will become much easier to get funding and support for further research.

One organisation that has been campaigning for many years for this is the Multidisciplinary Association for Psychedelic Studies (MAPS). Although MAPS focuses mainly on research into treating conditions like post-traumatic stress disorder and cluster headaches, it recognises the value of psychedelics outside the medical setting. One of its founders, Rick Doblin, has suggested that perhaps the way to make these sorts of drugs available in the future would be to issue [†]a licence once someone has participated in a workshop, or perhaps passed a test, to ensure that they know how to use them safely. Licensed users would understand the importance of being in the right frame of mind and environment, and the dangers and risks of a bad trip. Ideas like this are certainly something to consider, given the enormous potential of psychedelics to improve people's lives.

Notes

Page

248 (Figure 14.1),• *Neural correlates of the psychedelic state as determined by fMRI studies with psilocybin*, URL-171, Robin L. Carhart-Harris et al, PNAS, vol. 109 no. 6 2138–2143, February 7th, 2012

249 a theory that the stories of magic and devils reported by the girls of Salem• *Egotism: The Satan loosed in Salem?*, Linnda Caporeal, Science (192), April 2nd 1976

249 *"was seized by a peculiar sensation of vertigo and restlessness ... In a dreamlike state, I left for home ... With my eyes closed, fantastic pictures of extraordinary plasticity and intensive colour seemed to surge towards me."*• *LSD: my problem child*, Albert Hofmann, McGraw-Hill Book Company, 1980

249 *"I lost all control of time*• As above.

250 they recorded that they found themselves taking their schizophrenic patients' accounts of their illness more seriously• *Hofmann's Potion: The Early Years of LSD*, Connie Littlefield, URL-120, 2002

251 The LSD trials at Saskatchewan• As above.

252 outbreak of insanity in the French town of Pont-Saint-Esprit in 1951• *A terrible mistake*, Hank Albarelli, Trine Day, 2009

252 Leary first tried psilocybin, the active ingredient in magic mushrooms, and he soon began experimenting with LSD as well• *Hofmann's Potion: The Early Years of LSD*, Connie Littlefield, URL-120, 2002

254 "hearing voices"• *Schizophrenia,* National Institute of Mental Health , URL-118.

254 an edition of Spiderman in 1971• *The Amazing Spiderman issues #96–98,* Stan Lee, Marvel Comics, May–July 1971

255 five other studies that have found LSD helps people overcome alcoholism• *Lysergic acid diethylamide (LSD) for alcoholism: a meta-analysis of randomized controlled trials,* Teri S. Krebs and Pal-Orjan Johansen, Journal of Psychopharmacology, 2011

256 cluster headaches self-medicate with psychedelics• *Will Harvard drop acid again?,* Peter Bebergal, URL-121, June 9th 2008

256 use in problem solving• *LSD – The Problem Solving Psychedelic,* PG Stafford and BH Golightly, Award Books, 1967

258 Francis Crick• *Nobel Prize Genius Crick was High on LSD when he discovered the secret of life,* Alun Rees, the *Mail on Sunday,* August 8th 2004

258 Kary Mullis• BBC Horizon – *Psychedelic Science – DMT, LSD, Ibogaine* – Part 5, BBC, 1997

258 polymerase chain reaction (PCR)• The polymerase chain reaction is used to "amplify" a small amount of DNA, to produce a larger quantity that makes testing possible or easier. It is used every day in every aspect of life sciences, including forensic investigation and medical diagnosis.

258 There are many other kinds of psychedelic drugs• *High Society,* Mike Jay, Thames & Hudson, 2010

260 few recorded incidents of people taking them accidentally• As above.

260 Valeda mushroom ceremony in Mexico• *Seeking the magic mushroom,* Robert Gordon Wasson, Life Magazine, June 10th 1957

262 a licence once someone has participated in a workshop, or perhaps passed a test, to ensure that they know how to use them safely• *Will Harvard drop acid again?,* Peter Bebergal, URL-121, June 9th 2008

15 The War on Drugs, and drugs in war

[†]*"Public enemy number one in the United States is drug abuse. In order to fight and defeat this enemy, it is necessary to wage a new, all-out offensive."* **Richard Nixon**, 1971.

In 1971, President Nixon gave a speech in which he declared that the USA was facing a "national emergency", and that drug addiction was "public enemy number one". This was the beginning of the "War on Drugs", a term coined as a reference to President Lyndon Johnson's "War on Poverty", (which has been about as unsuccessful as the "War on Drugs" and the "War on Terror" which followed it). The word "war" in this case was oddly appropriate, as the "drug abuse emergency" Nixon referred to was largely taking place amongst the US Army in Vietnam, where drug-taking was very prevalent. To understand the origin of Nixon's policies, we first need to look at a little history of this other "war on drugs" – how drugs have been used in war zones over recent centuries.

The other "war on drugs"

High-strength drugs have been a common feature of battle zones, start-ing with the use of gin by William of Orange's soldiers (and hence the phrase "Dutch courage"). Large quantities of morphine were made avail-able to soldiers in the Franco-Prussian and American Civil wars and were especially popular after the invention of the hypodermic syringe. Cigarettes were popularised by Turkish troops in the Crimean War and the expansion of the cigarette market was helped by the inclusion of cigarettes in ration packs in the two World Wars. A common effect of fighting in a war is post-traumatic stress disorder (PTSD) – which was known as "shell shock" in the World War I and "battle fatigue" in World War II. In the past, PTSD was treated with bromides and barbiturates, and trials are currently being conducted on the use of psychedelics and ecstasy to treat the disorder in soldiers. For many veterans past and present, however, the most reliable and accessible drug for dealing with the trauma of war has been alcohol. The twentieth century also saw the widespread use of stimulants to enhance performance on the battlefield, though it's arguable they may have been more of a hindrance than a help. (See box *Amphetamines and war* below.)

What's surprising to us today is not so much that these drugs were used in the context of war, but how widely known and accepted the practice was. During World War I, [†]Harrods sold gift packs containing cocaine and heroin with the tag-line *"a welcome present for our friends at the front"*, and during World War II there were advertisements encouraging people to *"send your boys Benzedrine"*. (Benzedrine is an amphetamine.) But whereas these drugs were dispensed or approved by military doctors, for performance enhancement and pain relief, the use of drugs by USA troops in Vietnam was unsanctioned, and mostly involved cannabis and opiates. [†]Around 50% of the troops tried opium and heroin, half of whom started showing signs of addiction; two thirds of the troops used cannabis regularly. What frightened the Nixon administration was the prospect of large numbers of addicts flooding back into civilian life as the war settlement was negotiated and the military demobilised. This, coupled with the highly-public use of cannabis and psychedelics by the flower power counter-culture, created the cultural background to the War on Drugs. In fact, most of the USA soldiers using opioids in Vietnam stopped easily once back in the safety of the USA.

Amphetamines and war

The use of drugs has historically been common in the military, with soldiers trying to survive physical danger and lack of sleep and cope with the psychological trauma of experiencing and inflicting violence. Today, Western armies have strict drug-testing regimes because of concerns that drugs will impact on soldiers' health and performance in the theatre of war. But there was a time when the widespread use of certain substances, particularly stimulants like amphetamine, were thought to hold the key to military superiority. This theory was tested to its limit during World War II.

Stimulants is the general term for a class of drugs that includes amphetamine, methamphetamine, and derivatives like modafinil and Ritalin. Amphetamine is a synthetic derivative of ephedrine – a stimulant compound found in various species of Ephedra plant, which have been part of Chinese medicine for thousands of years. Ephedrine was isolated in 1885 and amphetamine synthesised two years later, but it wasn't until the 1930s that it found a medicinal purpose, as an inhaler for asthmatics. It was sold first of all as a liquid preparation under the name Benzedrine, and later produced in pill form.

Amphetamine was the drug of choice for the Allies – [†]the British alone used 70 million amphetamine tablets over the course of World War II – which helped soldiers to stay awake and alert for long hours. The Germans, meanwhile, were dosed up on Pervitin, a pill form of methamphetamine. Today, the most widely-used form of methamphetamine is the freebase that can be smoked, commonly known as "crystal meth" because it looks like a crystalline rock. (Crystal meth has a similar relationship to amphetamine as crack cocaine to cocaine powder.) When methamphetamine is smoked, it is more powerful and addictive than amphetamine partly because it reaches the brain faster. However, even when both drugs were being taken orally as pills in World War II, the methamphetamine in Pervitin worked faster than the amphetamine in Benzedrine, giving bigger highs, more energy, and helping soldiers stay awake for longer – at least at first.

As the war progressed, it became clear that these drugs were addictive, and that any performance improvement they created was at best short lived; the advantage of increased energy was soon outweighed by side-effects, including irritability, restlessness, inability to focus, and psychosis. Another classic side-effect was the development of *stereotypy* – involuntary, repetitive movements or behavioural patterns that impair the person's cognitive flexibility and judgement. This could be extremely dangerous when flying planes or handling guns and weapons. Methamphetamine takes longer to be processed by the body so its side-effects last longer, as well as being more severe, and it produces more withdrawal exhaustion when it is stopped. [†]After 1941, Pervitin was dispensed with much more discretion. (It's possible that the choice of drug affected outcomes of battles such as the North African campaign, because the amphetamine-taking Allies were more likely to able to sleep during the day, while the methamphetamine-using Germans couldn't rest and couldn't think as flexibly.)

In conventional warfare, most Western militaries are now very strict about the use of drugs, even when soldiers are off duty. The USA army does, however, use the wakefulness-promoting agent modafinil in the Middle East; this is a genuine performance enhancer in that its side-effects don't outweigh its benefits over the long-term, and it has few withdrawal effects. The British military remains sceptical of it, and it's possible that British soldiers have been disadvantaged because they've been unable to stay awake in conditions where the drug would have been beneficial.

Amphetamines are also given to soldiers in non-government armies under conditions where unpredictable behaviour rather than strict discipline are seen as advantages, such as in unconventional war zones. [†]Child soldiers in Sierra Leone, for example, are often dosed up on amphetamines before they fight, to make them more violent and less fearful – and the militias who recruit them probably think children who develop amphetamine psychosis make better soldiers. Disarming and rehabilitating these children is especially difficult as many are also dealing with drug addiction when they try and re-enter civilian life.

The aims of the War on Drugs

Nixon's speech came ten years after the [†]1961 *UN Single Convention on drugs*. This had already set the tone of the debate as a moral battle in which the use of certain sorts of drugs for pleasure was an evil to be eradicated, rather than a public-health issue to be managed. To quote the Convention Document, those who made the legislation were:

- Concerned with the health and welfare of mankind.
- Recognising that addiction to narcotic drugs constitutes a serious evil for the individual and is fraught with social and economic danger to mankind.
- Conscious of their duty to prevent and combat this evil.

What Nixon did was take this moralising approach to drugs – that they were inherently evil, and that our aim should be a "drug-free world" – and instigate a highly-combative set of policies in order to achieve it. The war would be fought on two fronts, (a) cutting off the supply of drugs by destroying crops and seizing the manufactured products, and (b) reducing demand through education and the threat of criminal sanctions. It was hoped that supply-side measures would drive up prices, reducing the amount being consumed on the street, and that demand-side measures would reduce the market and profits to be made.

Forty years ago, we knew much less about the harms done by psychoactive substances, about how addiction worked, or what the dynamics of the drugs trade were. Although the War was not framed in terms of harm reduction, it was thought that the combination of lower supply and demand would *automatically* minimise harm. Nowadays, a common view is that harm reduction and being "tough on drugs" are mutually exclusive. However, when the War on Drugs was initiated, it was viewed as a set of policies "concerned with the health and welfare of mankind", seeking to improve health and well-being across the world.

The War on Drugs has been very costly, and it would seem logical to try and work out whether it has achieved its stated aims. When we try and evaluate the success of these policies, we need to ask three questions. (A) Has the War on Drugs reduced supply? (B) Has it reduced demand? And (C) has it minimised harm?

Drugs – without the hot air, David Nutt

A. Has the War on Drugs reduced supply?

In 2003, †The No. 10 Downing Street Strategy Unit produced an analysis of the harm caused by heroin and crack use in the UK, and gave a comprehensive overview of the supply-side strategies employed in the War on Drugs. These interventions have ranged from trying to reduce the production of the raw materials in source countries, to targeting street dealers in the UK. The aim has been to restrict the supply of drugs to consumers, so price rises and users consume less. The report evaluated the effectiveness of each of these strategies in turn.

The first intervention the report examined, at the top of the supply chain, is trying to reduce the quantities of coca leaf and opium grown. This can be done in three ways – destroying the crops and compensating farmers, destroying crops and not compensating farmers, and encouraging viable alternatives. Uncompensated destruction is the cheapest option, but creates social tension and consigns farmers to grinding poverty, and thus into the arms of anti-capitalist revolutionary groups. Compensated destruction is expensive and can end up incentivising farmers to grow more of the illicit crops rather than shifting to other sources of income. The third option is the most successful, the No. 10 Strategy Unit analysis concluded, and has made a significant difference in countries like Thailand and Pakistan, but it is expensive and requires the development of good governance. Since the arrival of drug money often corrupts governments, and turns them into "narcostates", it is extremely difficult to create viable alternative sources of income in countries where the drugs trade is well established.

Whatever the approach, the report pointed out that higher-up members of the drugs trade rarely suffer when supply-side interventions focus on farmers. Instead, the high-ups move to remote regions or different countries when attempts to control production start to take effect. Given the unequal terms of trade for most export commodities that small-scale farmers grow (such as coffee and sugar), it is never difficult for organisations with money to persuade or coerce them into switching to illicit crops. The report concluded that as long as there is a lucrative market for drugs in rich countries, and large numbers of easily exploited farmers in poor countries, it will be almost impossible for us to reduce substantially the quantity of drugs produced.

The next step is to try and seize consignments on their way to the UK, which is a better way of targeting the criminal organisations themselves. However, the Strategy Unit calculated that profit margins in the trade are so high – 26–58%, comparable with Gucci's profit margin of 30% – that we would need to make sustained seizures of around two-thirds of an organisation's product to have a good chance of making them go bust. Even when seizures are made on a scale that impacts on the cost of production, this often has little effect on street price. Traffickers usually cut their profits rather than passing on extra costs to wholesalers and dealers, and even when they do pass on the costs, the street price often does not increase because dealers tend to keep the price constant for their customers by reducing the purity (for cocaine) or selling the drug in smaller units (for heroin).

The report also questioned whether having a volatile street price for drugs is effective at reducing harm. Rising prices may reduce harm as users consume less per dose, but increases the risks from adulterants and can result in an increase in overdoses when the purity goes up again (which is particularly problematic with heroin where overdose often leads to death). The overall trend across the world for the last two decades, however, has been a steady decline in prices. Destroying crops in Colombia, or seizing even quite substantial quantities of illicit drugs as they travel to the UK, has not stopped users from being able to obtain them in whatever quantities they desire.

Once drugs arrive in the UK they are bought by wholesalers and distributors, and though police and customs do try to disrupt this part of the supply chain, it's very resource-intensive and difficult to make an impact as we know relatively little about this part of the supply chain. A far easier target is the thousands of street dealers. High-visibility policing can reduce their presence, and appease the public and media demands for action on drugs. But dealers are easily replaced and in any case removing a dealer removes only small quantities of drugs from the system. Disrupting retailer activity in the UK occupies a lot of police and court time, but doesn't stop people who want drugs getting their hands on them.

The final sort of supply-side interventions focus on money-laundering, but the Strategy Unit acknowledged that this is even harder to disrupt as it's shrouded in the secrecy of the offshore banking system.

The report concluded that, "despite interventions at every point in the supply chain, cocaine and heroin consumption has been rising, prices falling and drugs have continued to reach users." The drugs trade is not being harmed in any substantial way, and the drugs trade views government interventions simply as a cost of business rather than a threat to its viability. At best, these interventions may have been marginally successful at slowing the decline in price, but they have certainly failed to restrict the availability of drugs for those who want them.

B. Has the War on Drugs reduced demand?

	Opiates	Cocaine	Cannabis
1998	12.9 million	13.4 million	147.4 million
2008	17.35 million	17 million	160 million
% increase	34%	27%	8%

Table 15.1: Use of all illicit drugs has increased in the last decade.

Whether we're talking about problem drug users addicted to heroin and crack, or recreational users who occasionally smoke cannabis, a quick glance at official statistics (†Table 15.1) shows that the War on Drugs has failed to reduce demand. Although precise figures are hard to come by, the UN estimates of annual drug consumption across the world from 1998 to 2008 show a substantial increase for opiates, cocaine and cannabis, and there's no reason to believe that there have not been similar increases for amphetamines, ecstasy, and new designer drugs. The proud exhortation of the UN in 2001 that we'd have a drug-free world in 2010 has been exposed as a ridiculous rhetoric rather than a thought-out plan.

Although the War on Drugs is presented as a war on producers and dealers, in practice the focus has always been on the much easier target – the users. (Many of these are small-scale dealers themselves, selling to a handful of people in order to fund their own habits.) Addicts have a disease and are not in control of their actions, so putting them in prison is not only inhumane and extremely expensive, but it's completely useless in helping them manage their addiction. (†Only a fifth of the 50,000 problem drug users who end up in jail in the UK every year are given treatment.) Getting a criminal record or going to jail reduces the addicts' chance of being able to rebuild their lives even if they do stop using the drugs. Moreover the stress, boredom, and culture of prison creates more addicts, rather than incentivising them to give up. †About 20% of prisoners are addicted to opiates, and 7% try heroin for the first time in jail. Overall, targeting and imprisoning drug users does not reduce demand.

In general, criminal sanctions have very little influence on the prevalence of drug use in a population, which seems to be affected more by cultural trends, fashion and norms than the legal framework. †A comparative study of Australian states found that there was no relationship between how punitively the criminal justice system treated cannabis and levels of cannabis use, and this lack of correlation is replicated worldwide. Government-led education programmes, such as the †USA's Drug Abuse Resistance Education (DARE) programme (which also operates in the UK) has been found in some instances to *increase* drug use among participants in the short-term, probably because the children involved have developed an interest in the substances they've been told to "Just Say No" to. Over the long-term, research has found no difference between participants and non-participants, and †in 2001 the US Surgeon General placed the DARE programme in the category "Does Not Work".

Does criminalisation reduce the drug supply?

Locking up large numbers of people might be considered worthwhile if it reduced the supply of drugs to others. Is there any evidence that this is the case? The problem is, the people that go to prison are the wrong ones. Across the world, †two million drug offenders are currently in jail – about a quarter of the total prison population. Most are imprisoned for non-violent crimes, and most are at the very bottom of the drugs trade – small-scale dealers, user-dealers, drug mules who take small quantities over borders, and those convicted for possession.

On the rare occasions that people higher up within criminal organisations are arrested, bribes and expensive lawyers can usually secure their release. And even when drug cartels are successfully smashed by law enforcement agents, this doesn't reduce harm, and may even increase it as competing groups battle over the new markets. As long as the demand remains, somebody will produce the drugs to meet it. [†]Small-scale seizures and imprisoning those at the very bottom of the supply chain has no dampening effect on the business.

C. Has the War on Drugs minimised harm?

The short answer is, no. In fact it has done the opposite: it has increased harm for pretty much everyone. This is a well known amongst policy-makers, though rarely openly acknowledged. The most controversial aspect of the No. 10 Strategy Unit Report was its attempt to evaluate whether supply-side interventions might have been successful at harm reduction, pointing out that *"current policies are underpinned by an assumption that reducing drug availability and increasing price reduces harm."* The report heavily implied that this assumption was false, since there is little evidence that (a) supply-side seizures are able to reduce availability and increase price or (b) that overall levels of harm respond in any straightforward way to changes in price or availability where they do occur. [†]The report, unsurprisingly, was suppressed by the government, but released under the Freedom of Information Act and leaked to the media and is now available online. This is a common pattern: anything that tries to measure or evaluate the success of the War on Drugs inevitably finds that it has failed, so evaluation and measurement are either suppressed, or not carried out in the first place.

In terms of demand-side interventions, some of this increase in harm has been intentional – primarily, the harm caused by criminalising millions of people around the world. But a great many other sorts of harm have been more or less accidental, perverse effects which although predictable were not intended by those who instigated the War. These "perverse effects" include:

1. Increasing the spread of infectious disease.
2. Causing terminally ill people to die in agony.
3. Increasing instability and unaccountability in financial systems.
4. Holding back research on new medicines.
5. Increasing levels of drug-related violence and crime.
6. Increasing the number of users by forcing them to become dealers.
7. Bringing the law into disrepute; allowing discriminatory policing.
8. Diverting attention away from the dangers of alcohol and tobacco.

1. Increasing the spread of infectious disease

Injecting drug users are a group who are particularly vulnerable to health problems from blood-borne viruses such as hepatitis and HIV. Across the world, [†]3 million injecting drug users are living with HIV, and another 13 million are at risk of contracting it. This poses a public-health risk not only to the users themselves, but to their families, sexual partners, and others in society. Harm-reduction measures such as needle exchanges have been shown to reduce dramatically the prevalence of blood-borne viruses among drug users. However, some countries have taken the attitude that, since this group is using substances controlled under the international conventions of the War on Drugs, they shouldn't have access to clean needles to reduce their chances of becoming infected, or treatment if they do become unwell.

The situation is particularly bad in Russia, where the failure to implement needle exchange programmes or other harm reduction approaches when HIV appeared has resulted in one of the highest new infection rates in the world today – [†]about 60,000 new cases in 2009, according to the UN AIDS program. [†]Two thirds of these cases are linked to intravenous drug use, and many of the remainder are the result of sex with drug users. In some cities, antiretroviral medicines to treat AIDS are denied to drug users, speeding up their progression from HIV to AIDS.

There are other indirect health problems that result from this denial of healthcare to injecting drug users. Living in poverty for many years with low immunity and irregular or inadequate access to medication means that many of these people develop [†]"TurBo-HIV", contracting TB on top of the immunodeficiency virus. Many treatment programmes will only treat them for one health problem at a time, forcing them to choose between being treated for their addiction or for their TB. Since drug users' lives are often chaotic anyway, being unable to receive holistic care means that they often move between different treatment programmes, stopping and starting courses of different sorts of medication – exactly the circumstances that cause viruses to mutate. The result is one of the highest rates of multidrug-resistant TB in the world, a hazard to health that extends beyond the users themselves, affecting Russian society at large. This situation could largely have been prevented if injecting drug users had been viewed as sick patients requiring medical help; instead, the attitude fostered by the War on Drugs was that they were immoral people deserving punishment.

2. Causing terminally ill people to die in agony

The War on Drugs has caused a chronic lack of pain killers, particularly morphine, in around half the countries in the world. Strict controls in India, for example, mean that doctors can go to prison if a little as 1 mg of morphine goes missing, and in the Ukraine the approved government dose is only 7 mg a day, a tiny fraction of what would be prescribed in the UK for severe conditions. These controls, of course, are in place because of morphine's close similarity to heroin, which is one of the main targets of the War on Drugs. Morphine, like other opiates, does cause physical dependence and can lead to addiction, though it's rare for people who've had it administered for pain control within a medical setting to have psychological cravings when they stop.

While heroin is a harmful drug, it's perverse if trying to reduce its use forces many people with terminal cancers [†]to live the last months or years of their lives in agony, when an adequate supply of cheap morphine tablets would make them bearable. The palliative-care movement within the Indian state of Kerala has managed to relax the rules around the prescription of opiates, but in 27 other Indian states it remains almost impossible to provide morphine for those who need it most. (This is particularly galling as India is one of the world's biggest suppliers of opium, and morphine tablets cost only pennies to produce.) Campaigning groups such as Human Rights Watch have argued that freedom from pain should be considered a human right, and have compared the testimonies from terminal cancer patients without access to painkillers to the testimonies of those who have suffered torture. They continue to campaign to remove medical morphine from the War on Drugs.

3. Increasing instability and unaccountability in financial systems

The illicit drugs trade is the second largest in the world, second only to oil. The money involved – perhaps [†]£300 billion a year – is about 1% of the global economy, and operates almost entirely under the radar, untaxed and unregulated.

Drugs money is laundered through front companies and tax havens, and then integrated back into the mainstream banking system so that criminal organisations can have access to "legitimate funds". A number of different techniques are used, such as small-scale electronic transfers and false invoicing: it's been estimated that [†]in Panama there is a £1 billion gap every year between money entering and goods exported, with the difference plugged with the proceeds of various sorts of crime, primarily drug trafficking.

[†]Banks, in turn, are complicit in this process, failing to report or record suspicious activity, because some are controlled by criminal organisations, and perhaps also because offshore banking services depend on secrecy for tax evasion and avoidance. Exposing the activities of drug traffickers would expose the activities of other clients. Making it easier for large volumes of money to travel the world without any kind of accountability undermines governments and is dangerous for the financial system as a whole. There were many causes of the financial crisis which began in 2008, but a chief reason that the asset bubble in subprime housing was able to grow so large was that the people in charge of the banks had no idea where their money was coming from or where it was be-

Drugs – without the hot air, David Nutt

ing invested. In 2010, a single bank, †Wachovia, paid $160m to settle a US federal investigation into laundering of illegal drug money through Mexican currency exchanges. This included a $50m fine for failing to monitor money used for shipping 22 tons of cocaine. †Wachovia was unable to check about $400bn's worth of transactions to see if money was being laundered. For such huge sums to pass through a bank's system without raising comment shows a very worrying lack of concern for the law and transparency in financial transactions.

4. Holding back research on new medicines

When a drug becomes illegal, conducting experimental research on it is much more difficult. Researchers have to apply for special licences to synthesise or obtain samples, and go through excessively arduous processes about reducing the possible risks to those involved in the trials. Because pharmaceutical companies know that any drug with a chemical similarity to an illegal psychoactive substance is unlikely to be approved, they tend to avoid these areas of research altogether. The situation is particularly bad in the USA, where analogues are automatically illegal, but it's also problematic in the UK. This has held back research into the use of ecstasy in helping those with PTSD, into psychedelics for tackling addiction, and into cannabis for pain relief, and so on.

5. Increasing levels of drug-related violence and crime

As we discussed in chapter 10, the drugs trade is responsible for very high levels of violence and crime, both internationally and at home. Attempts to meet this head-on tend to make the problem worse: often it's †when a government says it's going to "crack down" on the illicit trade that violence worsens, as we've certainly seen in Mexico.

The criminal organisations that supply drugs are often involved in people-trafficking and modern slavery, and they actively work to corrupt and destabilise governments. †Al Qaeda is principally funded by opium and cannabis production, and †Mexican drug cartels are involved in kidnapping, counterfeiting and business extortion, as well as being responsible for tens of thousands of murders.

The corrupting effects of drug money have been seen most recently in the West African countries which have become the transit routes for cocaine travelling from South America to Europe. In an address in December 2007, UN Office on Drugs and Crime (UNODC) Executive Director Antonio Maria Costa described Guinea-Bissau as [†]*"under siege. The threat posed by drug traffickers is so great that the state is on the verge of collapse ... So much drug money flowing in so easily, is a true curse: it is perverting the economy and rotting society."* In 2010, the leaders of both the army and the navy were sanctioned for trafficking cocaine, showing that this corruption has reached to the highest levels.

In the UK, drug users commit a very high proportion of acquisitive crime. [†]85% of shoplifting and 80% of domestic burglary is committed by problem drug users, which is unsurprising considering that a heavy heroin habit costs £300 a week, and a bad crack addiction can cost over £500 a week. [†]There are over 300,000 problem drug users in the UK, but surprisingly, it is a hard-core of [†]30,000 who commit over half of all drug-related crime, costing the country £11 billion a year, or £360,000 each. Providing a methadone or heroin prescription for these people would cost a fraction of £360,000, but many users are afraid to begin treatment programmes because of the possibility that once the authorities know they use drugs, they will be targeted and imprisoned.

6. Increasing the no. of users by forcing them to become dealers

[†]In 1955, there were 57 registered heroin addicts in the UK. Most of these were under the medical supervision of their GP who helped to treat or manage their addiction. This option was then outlawed, as "public" opinion saw it as the state condoning a drug-using lifestyle. (The new UK coalition government is resurrecting this old rhetoric as it tries to save money and appease voters by stopping substitute prescribing – see page 167.) Today, there are estimated to be at least 300,000 registered addicts, with fewer than half going into treatment over the course of each year. While there were many social, demographic and technological changes fuelling this huge rise in the number of addicts, one was undoubtedly the fact that creating a black market for drugs simultaneously

Drugs – without the hot air, David Nutt

created drug "pushers" – people with an incentive to get others hooked on addictive drugs in order to make money. Many of the pushers were addicts themselves who had to buy heroin illegally, now that they no longer received heroin on prescription. They found small-scale dealing was the easiest source of funds, creating a kind of pyramid scheme where every addict created ten or more new ones. In fact, in 1955 the government was warned that this would be an effect of banning the drug, in an article published in *The Times* in 1955 entitled [†]*The Case for Heroin*. Over five decades later, they've certainly been proved right, and at last we have some [†]new trials of heroin-prescribing under way with promising results.

7. Bringing the law into disrepute; allowing discriminatory policing

In 2000, an enquiry led by [†]Viscountess Runciman produced a report into the policing of drugs in the UK, with a particular focus on cannabis. The report concluded that:

> "There can be no doubt that, in implementing the law, the present concentration on cannabis weakens respect for the law ... It gives large numbers of otherwise law abiding people a criminal record. It inordinately penalises and marginalises young people for what might be little more than youthful experimentation. It bears most heavily on young people in the streets in cities who are also more likely to be poor and members of minority ethnic communities. The evidence strongly indicates that the current law and its operation creates more harm than the drug itself."

The Runciman report also found evidence of political or discriminatory policing. Individual police officers were given a large degree of personal discretion about how strictly they enforced laws on cannabis. This let some police officers pursue other agendas, such as the control of young men from ethnic minorities by disproportionately prosecuting them for possession, as illustrated clearly by the official statistics on stop-and-search and court procedures. The Runciman report was pivotal in cannabis being downgraded from Class B to Class C, but the drug was re-graded shortly afterwards, and ten years on discriminatory policing continues. [†]People from black communities are 6 or 7 times more likely to be arrested if they're found with drugs than people from other ethnic groups, and 11 times more likely to be imprisoned. This sours the relationship between these communities and the police, normalises criminality, and was a significant factor in provoking the 2011 riots in London.

8. Diverting attention from the dangers of alcohol and tobacco

[†]Each year, tobacco kills 5 million people across the world, while [†]alcohol kills 1.5 million. By comparison, [†]illicit drugs kill around 200,000 people between them. Even taking into account the much smaller populations who use these drugs, in many cases they are considerably less deadly. Yet the levels of money and political will expended on trying to eradicate their use far exceeds the levels spent on public-health measures to reduce the harms of alcohol and tobacco. In addition, the small expenditure on reducing alcohol and tobacco consumption is counteracted by advertising from the drinks and tobacco industries which associate these drugs with health and beauty. Politicians often say that criminalisation is designed to "send a message" that the use of certain drugs is unacceptable because of the harm they cause to individuals and society. Unfortunately, the resultant message perceived by many millions of people around the world is that alcohol and tobacco are acceptable – and we all pay the price for that.

Why are we still at war?

After forty years, thousands killed, millions imprisoned, and [†]$1 trillion spent ([†]or $2.5 trillion depending on who you ask), we are still no closer to controlling either the supply- or demand-side of the illicit drug trade. Government interventions on the supply side are seen as a cost of business, like a tax rather than a serious threat; and the billions spent on DARE programmes and locking up users haven't stopped the inexorable rise of drug use in most parts of the world. In its own terms, the War on Drugs has failed, and the evidence shows it was also the wrong strat-

Drugs – without the hot air, David Nutt

egy for harm reduction. The intentional and perverse effects of the war have spread disease, held back medical research, brought the law into disrepute, and ruined the lives of millions.

But still our politicians keep fighting, at least while they hold power. [†]Mo Mowlam, who had been responsible for Tony Blair's anti-drugs policies, called for full legalisation after she'd left politics in 2002. Former Home Secretary [†]Bob Ainsworth spoke out about decriminalisation when safely out of the Cabinet and in opposition. Former presidents [†]Bill Clinton and Jimmy Carter criticised the War on Drugs in a recent documentary. [†]Jimmy Carter wrote an article entitled *Call Off the Global Drug War* in *The New York Times*, and in November 2011, along with many Nobel prizewinners, international statesmen, and other public figures, wrote a public letter entitled [†]*The Global War On Drugs Has Failed: It Is Time For A New Approach*. And in 2002, an ambitious UK backbencher called David Cameron said in a debate in the House of Commons [†]*"drugs policy has been failing for decades"*. Yet now that he's Prime Minister, Cameron talks just as "tough on drugs" as every other politician, and Obama, while supporting having a more open debate on drugs policy, always takes pains to make it clear he himself is absolutely committed to prohibition.

It seems impossible for current politicians to talk about anything other than outright prohibition – and since by almost every meaningful measure their policies are unsuccessful, they keep changing what they're measuring, emphasising the amount of money spent on law enforcement, the number of seizures made or the number of people they've arrested. But this makes a mockery of the whole idea of evidence-based policy. It is clear from the evidence that these are the wrong measures: if they've had any success at all, the politicians should be talking about declining numbers of users, decreased supplies on the street, or the reduction of harm.

Our politicians have backed themselves into a corner. In making the "tough on drugs" stance the only electorally-viable policy, and attacking anyone who proposes an alternative, they are forced to ignore the evidence all around them and the solutions that follow from seeing the world as it is, not as we pretend it is to fit in with a given political view point. This may be an easy vote winner at election time, but in the longer term it's bad for democracy, bad for science, and bad for the millions of casualties around the world affected directly and indirectly by this un-winnable War.

What are the alternatives?

If you criticise the War on Drugs, the stock media response is to accuse you of wanting to see heroin "on the supermarket shelves". This is a ridiculously-reductive response to the wide range of options available for dealing with drugs once prohibition stops being the only policy that can be considered. For a start, there is a big difference between legali-sation and decriminalising possession. In Portugal, heroin, cocaine and cannabis remain illegal, but possession of small amounts doesn't carry any criminal sanctions, like minor traffic offences in the UK. Decrimi-nalisation allows countries to focus on harm-reduction strategies while staying within the terms of the UN Single Conventions, but leaves all the supply-side problems intact. If we wanted to go further and make cer-tain drugs legally available, †there are lots of alternatives to unregulated sales:

- Making drugs available on prescription, so your doctor can moni-tor your use and help you through withdrawal if you wish to stop.
- Selling them from pharmacies, so the pharmacist can give advice on dose and possible side-effects. This idea could be developed to create a new profession specialising in recreational drugs, who are able to give counselling and intervene if they think someone is in danger of addiction.
- Licensed sales, so that only certain shops can sell them, under cer-tain conditions and at certain times.
- Licensed premises for consumption on site, like pubs or the Dutch cannabis cafes. These licences could be exclusive, so that a place which is allowed to sell ecstasy can't sell alcohol, for example, and licensees could be partially responsible for the behaviour of their customers. The Dutch coffee shops that sell cannabis are not only

Drugs – without the hot air, David Nutt

banned from selling alcohol, but also don't allow tobacco smoking on the premises.

- Membership-based licensed premises, where users have to be registered, and consumption can be monitored and controlled. Although we don't currently use this for drugs, it's similar to the model we've adopted for casinos, and in Spain a similar scheme for cannabis use seems to be working well.

The point is, there *are* a lot of alternatives. We don't have to choose a single option and apply it to every drug which is currently prohibited. We can decriminalise possession of small amounts for personal use without making all – or even any – drugs legal. We can treat addicts with dignity and respect and help them reduce the chaos of their lives without allowing dangerous substances to be aggressively advertised as alcohol is today. We can support poor coca and opium farmers while still trying to break the power of the criminal gangs that exploit them. We could do all sorts of things, weighing up the harms and benefits of different policies, learning from the experiences of other countries, and having reasoned debates about what the evidence shows and what we think that means we should do. But none of this is possible while the War on Drugs continues.

Comparing the harms of smoking cannabis with going to prison

Even though UK police officers often choose not to arrest or prosecute people when they're caught with cannabis, it remains the most common illicit drug to come before the courts because it's by far the most commonly used. Smoking cannabis and taking other drugs is a unique type of crime because it's a crime against yourself – the state has decided that the harms are so great you should be penalised, even to the point of imprisonment, to protect you from it. This only makes sense as a harm-reduction measure if taking cannabis is considerably more harmful than going to jail. The main concerns people have about cannabis are that: it causes mental-health problems; it's a gateway to other sorts of more harmful drugs; it might impair your career; it can lead to addiction; and it imposes economic costs on society. Let's compare for a moment these harms done by smoking cannabis and the harm done by going to prison.

Cannabis can certainly cause mental-health problems. As discussed in chapter 5, when I was on the ACMD we calculated that around [†]one in 5000 cannabis users will develop schizophrenia as a result of using the drug, and more will suffer short-term psychotic symptoms and depression. There is a risk, but it's relatively low. Going to prison on the other hand, is associated with very high levels of stress and depression. [†]Prisoners are about 10 times more likely to commit suicide than the general population, and [†]about 40% of men and 60% of women have some form of neurotic disorder. (Although these conditions may have preceded going to jail, making it difficult to establish cause-and-effect, these confounding factors are also true for cannabis.) Imprisoning people for using cannabis is clearly not going to protect their mental health.

Another common concern is that cannabis will act as a "gateway" to other more harmful substances. While it's true that most people who become addicted to heroin and crack have used cannabis, their first drug experiences tend to be alcohol and tobacco, so it's arguable that these are as much of a gateway to hard drug use. (Also, the vast majority of cannabis users never take heroin or crack.) Of course, because cannabis is illegal, obtaining it does put users in contact with dealers who might try to sell them other substances. The Dutch cafe "coffee shop" model for cannabis was set up largely to allow their young people to obtain the drug without coming into contact with dealers, who naturally want users to take more addictive and profitable drugs. The Dutch model was a logical and bold experiment in social drugs policy, which has worked extremely well. The Netherlands has some of the lowest levels of heroin use in Europe, showing that separating the supply-side can prevent cannabis use leading to hard drugs.

Drugs – without the hot air, David Nutt

If anything, prison is the biggest gateway of all, being awash with drugs and having very little in the way of other sorts of stimulation or sources of pleasure. Opiate use is particularly high, and 7% of prisoners say they first tried heroin in jail. The fact that Justice Secretary †Ken Clarke has been talking about "drug-free wings" in prisons is an open acknowledgement of the fact that even in the state's most tightly controlled spaces of all we still can't control the supply of drugs. In fact, attempts to deter substance abuse through drug testing in prisons is actually making this gateway effect more severe. Cannabis and its breakdown products can be detected in urine for weeks, whereas heroin clears from the body much faster. Testing positive for drugs can result in an increase in sentence, so prisoners have found a way to reduce the likelihood of being caught: use heroin instead of cannabis. Far from protecting them, imprisoning cannabis users will make them more likely to start using hard drugs.

It's unlikely that anyone's career is seriously impaired these days by admitting that they've tried drugs. Many of our MPs feel they can acknowledge cannabis use now, and Obama has even admitted to having taken cocaine, though British politicians have yet to be so honest. Although heavy use and addiction disrupts working life, low levels of cannabis consumption seem quite compatible with it, and may even be beneficial for some creative people. Prison, in contrast, is definitely bad for your career. †Research by the Department of Work and Pensions has found that the unemployment rate of ex-offenders is over 50%, and having a criminal record of any sort makes rejection probable for around 50% of job vacancies.

We say that someone is addicted when they keep repeating behaviour despite adverse consequences. About †10% of cannabis users become dependent, exposing themselves to health risks from heavy use, and falling behind at school or under-performing at work because they spend so much time intoxicated. Although it's hard to make a direct link between addiction to a drug and criminal behaviour, reoffending could be seen as comparable to addiction because even though someone's life has been harmed by committing crime they still end up repeating criminal behaviour. Ministry of Justice figures in 2010 showed that [†]50% of prisoners re-offend, in large part because when they leave prison they find it so hard to get a job or housing, which are the two most important factors in helping people stay away from crime. Imprisoning people for cannabis use is likely to get them caught up in a cycle of crime far more damaging that being addicted to the drug.

Finally, there's the issue of economic cost. While the economic burden of cannabis use is hard to calculate, it must be far lower than the [†]£38,000 it costs to keep somebody in prison for a year, and support them afterwards when they're unemployed or suffering mental-health problems. Imprisoning cannabis users places a huge burden on the police and courts, far greater than the drug itself.

So, prison is worse for people's mental health, more likely to lead to hard drug use, more likely to ruin someone's career, more likely to lead to a cycle of destructive behaviour, and is far more expensive for society than cannabis: imprisoning people for using cannabis increases harm, rather than reducing it. An alternative model for punishing those caught in possession of cannabis is the "Cameron approach". When [†]David Cameron was caught with the drug at Eton, he was made to write out hundreds of lines of Latin; there are certainly thousands of young people across the UK whose lives would be immeasurably improved if this became public policy.

Notes

Page

264 "Public enemy number one in the United States is drug abuse• *The Nation: The New Public Enemy No.1*, URL-122, June 28, 1971

265 Harrods sold gift packs containing cocaine and heroin• *Can we imagine a Britain where all drugs are legal?*, Mark Easton, URL-123, December 16th 2010

265 Around 50% of the troops tried opium and heroin• *Narcotic use in Southeast Asia and afterward: An interview study of 898 Vietnam returnees*, LN Robins, JE Helzer, DH Davis, Archives of General Psychiatry, 32(8), 955–961, 1975

266 the British alone used 70 million amphetamine tablets over the course of World War II• *Concepts of Chemical Dependency*, Harold E Doweiko, Cengage Learning, 2009

267 After 1941, Pervitin was dispensed with much more discretion• *Psychotherapy in the Third Reich: the Göring Institute*, Geoffrey Cocks, New Brunswick, NJ, 1997. Orders were given that Pervitin was to be kept "under lock and key" once side effects were recognised by military doctors.

267 Child soldiers in Sierra Leone, for example, are often dosed up on amphetamines before they fight• URL-156.

267 1961 *UN Single Convention on drugs*• Office of Drugs Control, URL-22, 1961

269 The No. 10 Downing Street Strategy Unit produced an analysis of the harm caused by heroin and crack use• *Strategy Unit Drugs Report Phase One – Understanding the Issues*, URL-124, May 12th 2003

271 Table 15.1• Reproduced from p4 of *War on Drugs: Report of the Global Commission on Drugs Policy*, URL-125, June 2011

272 Only a fifth of the 50,000 problem drug users who end up in jail in the UK every year are given treatment• *Strategy Unit Drugs Report Phase One – Understanding the Issues*, URL-124, May 12th 2003

272 About 20% of prisoners are addicted to opiates, and 7% try heroin for the first time in jail• *Compendium of Reoffending Statistics*, URL-127, May 10th 2011

272 A comparative study of Australian states found that there was no relationship between how punitively the criminal justice system treated cannabis and levels of cannabis use• *The impact of cannabis decriminalisation in Australia and the United States*, Eric Single, Paul Christie and Robert Ali, Drug and Alcohol Services Council South Australia, URL-128, 1999

272 USA's Drug Abuse Resistance Education (DARE) programme• *Youth illicit drug use prevention: DARE long-term evaluations and Federal efforts to identify effective programs*, United States General Accounting Office, URL-129, January 15th 2003

272 in 2001 the US Surgeon General placed the DARE programme in the category "Does Not Work"• *Youth violence: A report of the US Surgeon General* (chapter 5), David Satcher, URL-130, 2001

272 two million drug offenders are currently in jail – about a quarter of the total prison population• *After the War on Drugs – Options for Control*, Transform Drugs Policy Foundation, URL-131, February 2006

273 Small-scale seizures and imprisoning those at the very bottom of the supply chain has no dampening effect on the business• *Strategy Unit Drugs Report Phase One – Understanding the Issues*, URL-124, May 12th 2003

273 The report, unsurprisingly, was suppressed by the government, but released under the Freedom of Information Act and leaked to the media and is now available online• *No 10 Strategy Unit Drugs Project: Phase 1 Report: "Understanding the Issues"*, Transform, URL-132, accessed December 10th 2011

274 3 million injecting drug users are living with HIV, and another 13 million are at risk• *Injecting Drug Use and HIV*, UNAIDS, URL-133, accessed December 12th 2011

274 about 60,000 new cases in 2009• *Inadequate Fight Against Drugs Hampers Russia's Ability to Curb HIV*, Michael Schwirtz, URL-134, 16th January 2011

274 Two thirds of these cases are linked to intravenous drug use, and many of the remainder are the result of sex with drug users• *Russia's HIV care must centre on drug users*, Maria Golovanevskaya, URL-135, January 26th 2011

275 "TurBo-HIV", contracting TB on top of the immunodeficiency virus• *TurBoHIV*, Timur Islamov Charitable Foundation, URL-136, 2010

275 to live the last months or years of their lives in agony,• *The Pain Project*, Al Jazeera, URL-137.

276 £300 billion a year – is about 1% of the global economy• *After the War on Drugs – Options for Control*, Transform Drugs Policy Foundation, URL-131, February 2006

276 in Panama there is a £1 billion gap every year between money entering and goods exported• *Strategy Unit Drugs Report Phase One – Understanding the Issues*, URL-124, May 12th 2003

276 Banks, in turn, are complicit in this process, failing to report or record suspicious activity•As above.

277 Wachovia, paid $160m to settle a US federal investigation into laundering of illegal drug money through Mexican currency exchanges. This included a $50m fine for failing to monitor money used for shipping 22 tons of cocaine• *How a big US bank laundered billions from Mexico's murderous drug gangs*, the *Guardian*, URL-138, April 3rd 2011

277 Wachovia was unable to check about $400bn's worth of transactions• *Wachovia to settle drug-money laundering case*, (Associated Press), URL-180, March 17th, 2010

277 when a government says it's going to "crack down" on the illicit trade that violence worsens, as we've certainly seen in Mexico• *Q&A: Mexico's drug related violence*, BBC, URL-139, August 26 2011

277 Al Qaeda is principally funded by opium and cannabis production• *Al Qaeda's drugs trade keeps them afloat during the economic crisis*, Sebastian Abbot, URL-140, October 16th 2008

277 Mexican drug cartels are involved in kidnapping, counterfeiting and business extortion• *The cartels behind Mexico's drug war*, Kazi Stastna, URL-141, August 28th 2011

278 *"under siege. The threat posed by drug traffickers is so great that the state is on the verge of collapse ... So much drug money flowing in so easily, is a true curse: it is perverting the economy and rotting society."•* *International conference on drug trafficking in Guinea-Bissau*, Antonio Maria Costa, URL-142, December 19th 2007

278 85% of shoplifting and 80% of domestic burglary is committed by problem drug users• *Strategy Unit Drugs Report Phase One – Understanding the Issues*, URL-124, May 12th 2003

278 There are over 300,000 problem drug users in the UK• *Tackling Problem Drug Use*, House of Commons Committee of Public Accounts, URL-143, March 24th 2010

278 30,000 who commit over half of all drug-related crime, costing the country £11 billion a year• *Strategy Unit Drugs Report Phase One – Understanding the Issues*, URL-124, May 12th 2003

278 In 1955, there were 57 registered heroin addicts in the UK• *Heroin addiction in the United Kingdom (1954–1964)*, Thomas Bewley, British Medical Journal, URL-144, November 27th 1965

279 *The Case for Heroin•* *The Times*, June 14th, 1955

279 new trials of heroin-prescribing under way with promising results.• *Supervised injectable heroin or injectable methadone versus optimised oral methadone as treatment for chronic heroin addicts in England after persistent failure in orthodox treatment (RIOTT) : a randomised trial*, J Strang, N Metrebian, N Lintzeris et al, Lancet 375: 1885–95, 2010

279 Viscountess Runciman produced a report• *Drugs and the law*, Report of the Independent Inquiry into the Misuse of Drugs Act, Chairman Viscountess Runciman, URL-3, 2000

280 People from black communities are 6 or 7 times more likely to be arrested if they're found with drugs than people from other ethnic groups, and 11 times more likely to be imprisoned.• *Black people six times more likely to face drug arrest*, 172, Mark Townsend, the *Observer*, October 31, 2010; this *Observer* article discusses the analysis by Professor Alex Stevens of recent Ministry of Justice data, in his book *Drugs, Crime and Public Health: The Political Economy of Drug Policy*, Routledge, 2011

280 Each year, tobacco kills 5 million people across the world• *Why tobacco is a public health priority*, WHO, URL-145, accessed December 10th 2011

280 alcohol kills 1.5 million• *Global Status Report on Alcohol and Health*, WHO, URL-146, 2011

280 illicit drugs kill around 200,000 people between them• *Overview of global and regional drug trends and patterns*, UNODC World Drugs Report, URL-147, 2011

280 $1 trillion spent• *After 40 years, $1trillion dollars, US War on Drugs has failed to meet any of its goals*, Associated Press, URL-148, May 13th 2010

280 or $2.5 trillion• *The War on Drugs*, URL-178, Time Magazine, March 25th, 2009

281 Mo Mowlam• *'Legalise all drugs' – Mowlam*, BBC News, URL-149, April 28th 2002

281 Bob Ainsworth spoke out about decriminalisation when safely out of the Cabinet• *Can we imagine a Britain where all drugs are legal?*, Mark Easton, URL-123, December 16th 2010

281 Bill Clinton and Jimmy Carter criticised the War on Drugs in a recent documentary• *Breaking the Taboo*, (film), Fernando Grostein Andrade (director), 2011

281 Jimmy Carter wrote an article entitled *Call Off the Global Drug War* in *The New York Times•* URL-173, *The Opinion Pages*, June 16, 2011

281 *The Global War On Drugs Has Failed: It Is Time For A New Approach•* URL-176.

281 *"drugs policy has been failing for decades" •* Tory *Contender calls for more liberal drug laws*, Marie Woolf, URL-150, September 7th 2005

282 there are lots of alternatives to unregulated sales• *After the War on Drugs: Options for Control*, Transform, URL-151, February 2006

284 one in 5000 cannabis users will develop schizophrenia• *Cannabis: classification and public health*, ACMD, April 2008

284 Prisoners are about 10 times more likely to commit suicide• *Statistics 8: The Criminal Justice System*, Mind, URL-152, accessed December 10th 2011

284 about 40% of men and 60% of women have some form of neurotic disorder• As above.

285 Ken Clarke has been talking about "drug-free wings" in prisons• *Clark's vision: a return to Victorian-style prisons with hard work, discipline... and NO hard drugs*, Daily Mail Reporter, URL-153, October 14th 2010

285 Research by the Department of Work and Pensions• *Barriers to employment for offenders and ex-offenders*, Hilary Metcalf, Tracy Anderson and Heather Rolfe, URL-154, 2001

285 10% of cannabis users become dependent• *Cannabis: classification and public health*, ACMD, April 2008

286 50% of prisoners re-offend• *Compendium of Reoffending Statistics*, URL-127, May 10th 2011

286 £38,000 it costs to keep somebody in prison for a year• *Ken Clarke plans radical reform of the prison system*, Andrew Woodcock and Lucy Bogustawski, URL-155, June 30th 2010

286 David Cameron was caught with the drug at Eton, he was made to write out hundreds of lines of Latin• *Cameron – the rise of the new conservative*, Francis Elliott, Fourth Estate, 2007. *Exclusive: Cameron DID smoke cannabis*, Simon Walters, the *Daily Mail*, 181, February 12th, 2007

16 The future of drugs

The next 20 years hold great opportunities for drugs research and for improving our understanding of the brain. Developments in genetic sequencing technologies will make genotyping commonplace, and as we learn more about genetic variations and vulnerabilities, we'll be able to give people far more information on which to base their choices about drug-taking. Addiction research has developed rapidly in the last ten years, though how far it manages to progress in the years to come will depend largely on how well it's funded, and on a wider acceptance of the medical model of addiction amongst governments around the world. Potentially, however, we could see leaps forward in the development of pharmacological substitutes, antagonists to help people quit, and pharmacological aids in psychological treatments.

There are also risks, and difficult legal and ethical issues that will need to be addressed. We will almost certainly need to devise new commercial models for the development and distribution of drugs, and develop new forms of patent law. We will also face difficult social issues regarding political confidentiality and the protection of civil liberties. Here we'll look at some of the most promising avenues of research in the development of new drugs and treatments for addiction, and explore some predictions for the future.

Genetic sequencing

Within 20 years, it's likely that every child born in the UK will have their DNA sequenced at birth, perhaps with the data stored on a microchip under their skin. The primary purpose of this, from a therapeutic point of view, is to avoid many of the [†]thousands of deaths a year that occur when people have allergic reactions to the medication they're given in hospital. When someone is brought into an accident and emergency (A&E) department in 2030, they will have their microchip scanned and cross-referenced with a database of genetic variants that are known to predict problems with common medicines. This will save many lives.

(While this scanning sounds futuristic, in fact it's already done on a very small scale for one rare condition called [†]*phenylketonuria*. Every child is tested shortly after they're born. Blood is taken from a pinprick on their heel and tested for a genetic mutation that makes them unable to breakdown phenylalanine, the amino acid that dopamine and noradrenaline are made from. If untreated, people with this condition suffer a poisonous build-up of phenylalanine in the brain, leading to serious damage. Fortunately, testing for the genetic mutation means that we can put sufferers on a special diet avoiding high protein foods such as meat, eggs and milk – which contain phenylalanine – and they can lead relatively normal lives.)

How will genetic sequencing affect the way we use and abuse drugs outside the hospital setting? We know a little about how genetic variations can make people more vulnerable to the negative consequences of some drugs. A particular form of the serotonin transporter makes ecstasy users more likely to suffer depression, and variants on other genes can make you more likely to become dependent on alcohol, opiates or nicotine.

A gene which seems to affect the way many different drugs work is the one that determines how quickly we metabolise dopamine and noradrenaline, which are broken down by an enzyme called Catechol O Methyl Transferase (COMT). There are three genetic COMT types – about 25% of the population are "val-vals", who metabolise dopamine and noradrenaline quickly, another 25% are "met-mets", who metabolise them slowly, and the other 50% are "val-mets", who are somewhere in between.

When people are given a complex intellectual task such as a game where the rules keep changing, val-vals perform significantly worse than the other types (they make more errors); however, they [†]improve hugely when they're given stimulants, as shown in Figure 16.1. Val-mets, on

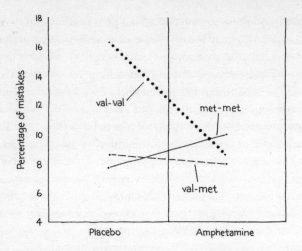

Figure 16.1: COMT type affects whether stimulants improve or worsen performance on complex intellectual tasks. The left shows performance on a placebo. The right shows performance on amphetamines: the val-vals (dotted line) perform better, the val-mets (dashed line) stay much the same, and the met-mets (solid line) perform worse.

the other hand, show very little change on stimulants, while met-mets perform worse. This is the principle behind prescribing stimulants for people with attention disorders, and although your COMT type doesn't seem to have a relationship to your likelihood of having ADHD, it does demonstrate that different people have different reactions to the same drugs.

We know a few other things about COMT type and drugs. [†]Val-vals are less pain sensitive, because they produce more endorphins when they are hurt. They may be more vulnerable to cannabis-induced psychosis. They also relapse faster when they try to give up smoking, probably because of low dopamine levels. All these traits together seem to make val-vals more exploratory, a kind of [†]"warrior" type who is more willing to take risks, while met-mets are the "worriers", who are naturally more cautious. One evolutionary theory behind the difference is that it was beneficial to human groups as we evolved to have both personality types in roughly equal measure.

Drugs – without the hot air, David Nutt

While these findings are interesting, our present knowledge is only the tip of the iceberg, partly because full genetic sequencing is currently so rare. There could be enormous potential benefits if millions of people share their genetic data and their experiences of illness, medication and drug taking via platforms like the internet. We'll be able to identify relationships between genes, illness, and drug effects; this will enable us to inform people about their vulnerabilities in ways that will make both therapeutic and recreational drug taking much safer. (That said, when it comes to complex behaviours like drug taking, genes are never deterministic. Having every known genetic vulnerability to smoking might increase your chances of addiction about three-fold – but not having those vulnerabilities will not protect you if you smoke persistently enough.)

What are the risks of genetic sequencing?

Widespread genetic sequencing will inevitably raise difficult questions. We'll need to establish how our genetic data should be used and shared, and how civil liberties and patient confidentiality can be protected without inhibiting research. And human genetics is a very sticky area in patent law. (Indeed, there was a race to sequence the human genome †between the publicly-funded Human Genome Project and the private company Celera Genomics. Had Celera won the race it's possible that they would have patented the entire thing, rather than allowing free redistribution and scientific use.) Understanding individual genetic variations might help us develop new medicines, but patent law will need to evolve to establish who has rights when someone's genetic material is being commercially exploited.

A famous case heard in 1990, †*Moore v Regents of the University of California*, revolved around whether a man called John Moore had the right to benefit financially from a cell line developed from his T lymphocytes, a type of white blood cell. The court ruled that he couldn't claim ownership of his own "discarded material", such as blood and tissue samples, and that the University were allowed to exploit the cell line commercially, as it was their invention. This sets quite a problematic precedent. On the one hand, it's better if people can't own their body parts, as that would mean that they could sell them for organ transplants or scientific research rather than donating them – but on the other hand, it seems unfair that an organisation or company should be allowed to make money out of other people's DNA in this way.

Genotyping will expose other ethical issues to do with risk, and how our predispositions relate to behaviour. We may end up with people claiming diminished responsibility for their actions because of their genetic code, or finding themselves uninsurable because they're considered at too great a risk of accidents or disease. As sequencing becomes more common, it will be very important that it's accompanied by education, and that there's a general understanding that genes are never the whole story: while genes might predict vulnerabilities, not having those genes certainly doesn't make us invulnerable. This is particularly true in terms of vulnerability to addiction, as it's a learned behaviour that requires voluntary repetition in order to become habitual. Knowing our genetic sequence might help us make better decisions, but genes alone aren't enough to protect us from the negative consequences of our own behaviour or the behaviour of others.

Treating addiction

Improving the treatment of addiction is one of the most promising lines of research. It's possible that within 20 years we will have far more effective therapies to prevent relapse, and even prevent addiction occurring in the first place. As our understanding of brain circuits develops, we may be able to predict from brain scans the extent to which an individual will like a particular drug, or how difficult they'll find it to stop. Someone who is found to have low numbers of dopamine receptors, for example, could be advised to avoid stimulants, as they're more likely to find them extremely pleasurable. We might even be able to treat such people with the sort of virus that has been used to grow more dopamine receptors in rats, protecting them from developing or relapsing into addiction.

A controversial topic that will almost certainly be part of the drugs debate in the next 20 years is the use of †vaccines to make drugs ineffective. We already use an immune-based approach to treat psychoactive drug use in a limited sense now – if people come to hospital with a cocaine overdose they're given antibodies that mop up the drug in the blood. This is a short-term treatment however, as it requires an intravenous infusion of the antibody, and the effect lasts just a few hours. In theory it should be possible to actively vaccinate someone against a drug, for example cocaine, so that when a person takes it the immune system is turned on to mop up the cocaine in the blood, stopping the drug from getting to the brain. This approach is theoretically possible for almost all substances, but currently the techniques to make the body raise its own immune response to a drug do not work as well as they do for vaccination against viruses such as polio. However, this is likely to change as more effort is put into vaccine development.

Vaccines for nicotine and cocaine are currently under clinical development, with a view to helping addicted users stop their habits. If this works then the question arises whether we could or should vaccinate people to protect them from developing an addiction in the first place, just as we do today with vaccines for polio and whooping cough. Even more controversial is the question of whether vaccines like this should be administered to children to immunise them against drug and alcohol use. Is it violating somebody's human rights to take away their choice to experience pleasure from a drug at some point in the future?

Learning and unlearning

Much of today's drugs research considers how pharmaceuticals can be used to make psychological treatments more effective. One area where this has had some success is in "unlearning", to help people overcome phobias. A phobia occurs when someone has a very powerful bad memory that overwhelms their rational reaction to a particular stimulus (such as a spider, or heights). To overcome the phobia they need to experience being in the presence of the feared object without feeling fear, and then make that memory more powerful than the phobic memory.

For example, a treatment devised for people with vertigo is to put them in a virtual-reality environment that gives them the sensation of being at a great height; at first, they're extremely afraid and panicky, but over several sessions their fear diminishes. What pharmacologists have developed is a drug that helps with forming the good, anxiety-free, memories.

Memories are made by changing the level in the brain of neurotransmitters, especially glutamate. The drug now in use for treatment of phobias is D-cycloserine which makes glutamate work better; when someone is given it during the virtual-reality sessions, they overcome their fearfulness more quickly. †Figure 16.2 compares treatment with D-cycloserine against treatment with a placebo.

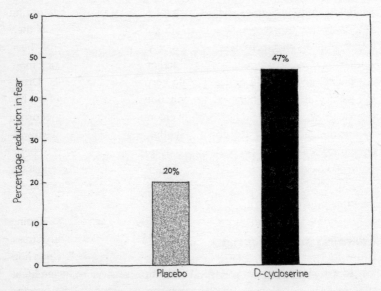

Figure 16.2: When people with a fear of heights were given D-cycloserine, three months after treatment their fear has reduced much more than if they were given a placebo.

We're now trying to work out how to apply these kinds of principles in treating addiction, which is also a learnt behaviour involving memory. The difficulty is that with illnesses such as phobias or post-traumatic stress disorder, the memories to be overcome are experienced as negative, so the patient has a big incentive to try to get better; in contrast, with addiction the memories laid down are profoundly positive, often the most positive experiences the patient has ever had. A big challenge in managing addiction is to help people overcome cravings by remembering the negative impacts of drug use instead of the positives. In the future, perhaps we'll use drugs like D-cycloserine to make somebody "phobic" to a drug they have abused, helping them to battle addiction.

New drugs research

There are a number of areas of research for new drugs. One interesting field is the use of psychedelics for treating addiction. Because of their legal status, the therapeutic properties of psychedelics have hardly been studied over the last 40 years, but this kind of research is becoming more acceptable now and will probably yield very interesting results. Drugs like psilocybin and ibogaine are not only non-addictive themselves, but seem to be effective at helping people overcome addictions to other drugs such as opiates, alcohol and nicotine. Synthetic analogues may be developed that have more predictable effects or minimise other sorts of harm – although it should be noted that psychedelics are already amongst the safest drugs we know of, particularly when administered within a therapeutic setting.

Almost all mental-health problems are prone to relapse; developing drugs that can reduce the factors that trigger relapse, particularly stress, is an important area of research. CRF and substance P are both stress hormones, which put you off your food and stop you sleeping when life is stressful. There is already some research showing that [†]alcohol craving can be reduced by using substance P antagonists, and in the future we may have similar or more effective drugs to reduce CRF as well. These would perform very similar functions to benzodiazepines or SSRIs prescribed for anxiety disorders, but because they would be targeting the stress hormone itself rather than GABA or serotonin, they might have fewer side-effects.

We may be able to make better recreational drugs as well. As discussed in chapter 6, I've done some research on replacing ethanol in "alcoholic" drinks with a safer alternative such as a reversible GABA-enhancer, and it may be that by 2030 that's what we'll all be drinking in the pub. An alternative approach is to modify alcohol itself to make it safer and more pleasant. We now know that alcohol works on a set of GABA receptors with different functions, and we have started to identify the different mechanisms involved. Receptors called Alpha-1 seem to control the sedative effect of alcohol, making you unsteady; [†]Alpha-5 receptors make you lose your memory; and we think Alpha-2 or Alpha-3 receptors make you feel relaxed and happy. In some very interesting studies, participants were given alcohol with an [†]inverse agonist that counters alcohol's effects on the Alpha-5 receptor. These participants performed much better on memory tests than those who had had alcohol on its own, showing it is possible to reverse at least one of the effects of alcohol with a drug. In principle, we could make alcohol safer by combining it with a range of inverse agonists that counter its negative effects on the other sorts of GABA receptors, too. It's likely, for example, that if we could find an inverse agonist for Alpha-1 you would be able to drink without becoming unsteady on your feet. Ideally, we would develop a version of alcohol which targets just Alpha-2 or 3, giving us all the sensation of relaxation and enjoyment without the negative effects.

The Brain Science, Addiction and Drugs Foresight programme

In the early 2000s, I became involved in the Brain Science, Addiction and Drugs project. This had been set up as part of the Foresight programme, which was introduced in the UK in 1992. The Foresight programme gathers expert opinions about the role science and technology might play in the issues we're going to face in the future. The program has looked at strategic issues such as changes in flooding risks, as well as the social implications of developments in fields such as fibre optics. As part of the Brain Science, Addiction and Drugs project I co-edited a book called

†*Drugs and the Future*, which gathered together some of our most up-to-date research, and explored the policy issues governments will need to face in the coming decades.

As part of the process we produced four different scenarios about what the UK might look like in 2025, both in terms of drugs policy and the wider social context. After much discussion, we decided that the two most important uncertainties were, firstly, whether decisions in the future would be based on the latest scientific evidence or on the latest social view, and secondly, whether the main focus for our use of drugs would be the enhancement of performance or the treatment of disease. From this we constructed a chart, and discussed the four scenarios that might occur at most extreme combinations of these two factors. We called these scenarios "high performance", "neighbourhood watch", "dispense with care", and "treated positively" (Figure 16.3). We then explored what these sessions might look like.

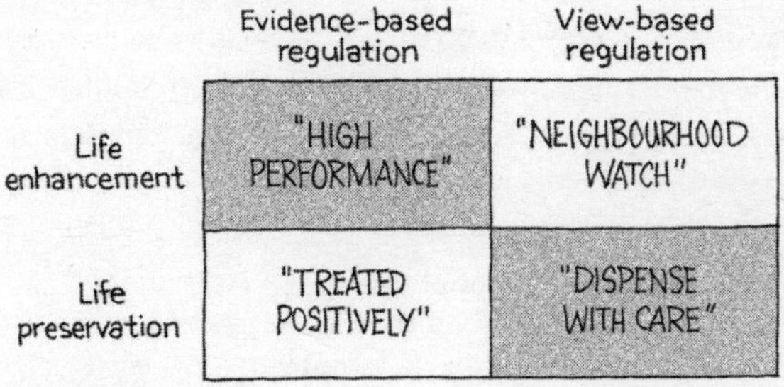

	Evidence-based regulation	View-based regulation
Life enhancement	"HIGH PERFORMANCE"	"NEIGHBOURHOOD WATCH"
Life preservation	"TREATED POSITIVELY"	"DISPENSE WITH CARE"

Figure 16.3: The chart used to construct our four scenarios.

1. The "high performance" scenario

In the "high performance" scenario, decisions are evidence-based, and the main focus for the use of drugs is the enhancement of performance. On this basis, it's expected that Britain has strong economic growth, in part because of its attractiveness to "knowledge nomads" (an elite class of highly mobile workers who migrate around the world moving between jobs in the knowledge economy). One of the things they like about Britain (in this hypothetical scenario) is our highly regulated, non-punitive approach to psychoactive substances, particularly cognition enhancers. Many recreational drugs are legal and available in high-quality forms to be consumed in special on-licence premises, although these are costly and there's a large black market in cheap generics from abroad. Problem drug-use with all its associated harms is on the decline.

The arguments that led the way towards legalisation and regulation of drugs were primarily economic, as it was felt that Britain was falling behind the Asian economies where cognition enhancers had become commonplace. The business community is very supportive of the legal use of drugs to improve performance at work, and by 2025 often contributes to their costs. Addiction is now seen solely as a medical problem, and treatments for it have become more effective because much investment has been put into research. The regulatory framework is grounded in a scientific appraisal of harms and benefits, and people regularly make use of genotyping technology to better understand the risks they're taking. This sort of predictive screening for vulnerabilities to particular drugs and addiction is common, and is credited with the large reduction in alcohol intake.

2. The "neighbourhood watch" scenario

In the "neighbourhood watch" scenario, decisions are based on social views rather than evidence, and the main focus for the use of drugs is the enhancement of performance. This version of the future is one of low economic growth, low consumer confidence and significant inequalities between different regions in the UK, particularly as a lot of power has been devolved to the regional level. Policy-making is largely based on moral views rather than scientific evidence. This combination has led to inconsistent, sometimes-incompatible policies from successive governments, following the prevailing dominant cultural views rather than rational appraisal of harm. Drug use is commonplace, despite the highly-punitive sanctions imposed by the criminal justice system, and addiction is seen as a moral failing that should be punished rather than treated as a medical disorder.

Drugs – without the hot air, David Nutt

This policy framework came about in response to a dramatic increase in drug use, particularly among the young and in poor communities, between 2010 and 2015, which prompted a moral backlash. Science was blamed for failing to contain the problem, but those leading the moral tide put most blame on the middle classes for casually consuming recreational drugs without regard for the misery their trade caused in the UK and abroad. A highly-punitive system involving drug testing at work and in schools, and heavy criminal sanctions, have led to a drop in drug use among the professional classes, and have slowed its spread elsewhere. However, the erosion of trust in science has meant that much research into the causes and treatment of drug abuse has been sidelined, and there's a growing recognition that to make the policy framework more sustainable science is required again. The UK has also failed to make any real headway in shutting down the international supply chain.

3. The "dispense with care" scenario

In the "dispense with care" scenario, decisions are based on social views rather than evidence, and the main focus for the use of drugs is the treatment of disease. By 2025, in this version of the future, one of the biggest problems facing the UK is the "demographic imbalance" – the worker-to-pensioner ratio has fallen to problematic levels. With 30% of the population over 60 (compared with about 20% in 2010), and a third of those over 70, there is a real shortage of skills in the labour market, and personal taxation is at its highest in decades. Given the spiralling costs of the healthcare system, there's been a decline in the standard of care, and the government has recently shifted all the costs of "self-inflicted" illness to the individual – so drug addicts, for example, can no longer receive treatment on the NHS.

Grey campaigners are a highly-mobilised political force and have lobbied very effectively for expensive life-preserving treatments (drugs to treat Alzheimer's, etc) to receive research investment and to be available to the public at large. However, because successive governments with low-taxation policies are repeatedly elected, this has led to unsustainable costs, and a degrading of public services, including the NHS.

Although steps have been taken to provide more funding for the NHS, decreasing its bill by refusing to treat self-inflicted illness may be indicative of future plans to reduce its remit.

4. The "treated positively" scenario

In the this final scenario, "treated positively", decisions are evidence-based, and the main focus for the use of drugs is the treatment of disease. Having invested heavily in addiction research, Britain is an acknowledged world leader in treating the disease, but there's a clear class divide: less well-educated people view addiction treatment with suspicion and exclude themselves from it. Cannabis was legalised for the terminally ill in 2014, and for other seriously-ill patients in 2018, but recreational use remains illegal, as with most other psychoactive substances. The research climate into possible therapeutic uses of drugs such as psychedelics, however, is far more supportive than it was in the past.

Although big pharmaceutical companies still play an important role in the market, smaller outfits have sprung up using "open source" genetic databases, producing precision treatments at much lower cost. This model has, of course, been copied in the illicit drug trade, and precision highs tailored to particular genotypes are about to hit the streets. The shift to smaller companies reflects a wider societal move towards smaller structures in the economy generally, accompanied by a cultural shift away from consumerism, and a more global outlook as we struggle with issues such as climate change and global equity. This cultural move towards higher quality of life has resulted in slower growth but better health outcomes.

What sort of future do we want?

As part of the Foresight project, we also consulted with stakeholders such as the pharmaceutical industry and the wider public. This threw up some new issues that will need to be resolved in coming years.

From the industry's point of view, getting drugs approved for mental-health disorders is now so difficult that many companies feel that the

Drugs – without the hot air, David Nutt

costs of developing them are simply not worth it. Investing $1 billion in a drug that may never come onto the market at all is a substantial risk, and means that companies often focus on making slight improvements to currently-approved drugs rather than exploring more radical options. While of course we need to protect the public from ineffective or harmful medicines, we also need to be able to experiment with new treatments. Perhaps the answer lies in smaller companies that can develop precision drugs, as suggested in the "treated positively" scenario; perhaps we need much better public funding; or perhaps we could move to the informed-consent model for drugs approval discussed in chapter 12. Whatever happens, we will have to think of alternatives if the big pharmaceutical companies stop developing the drugs that so many ill people rely on.

One of the chief concerns that came out of our consultation with the public, on the other hand, was the social implications of new medications. It was felt that an increasing focus on "normal" behaviour, which can be achieved by everyone with medication, will result in an excessively homogeneous society with little room for natural variations in personalities and mental capacities. There were also concerns that if cognition enhancers become commonplace, they could increase the economic divide between those who can afford them and those that can't.

Ultimately, a lot depends on what sort of future we *decide* that we want. What actually happens by 2025 will almost certainly involve elements from all four projected scenarios. Many of the factors that will shape our future are largely out of our control – including demographic shifts or needing to deal with climate change – but other factors will depend on the decisions our politicians make, and the role that we expect science to play in those decisions. It is unlikely that the pharmaceutical industry will ever have much of an interest in addiction treatment, for example, so if we want to find new ways of tackling the disease we'll need to ensure that public funding continues. Whatever happens, it's important that we begin the conversation about the society we want to create, and the role that drugs will play in that.

Notes

Page

292 thousands of deaths a year that occur when people have allergic reactions to the medication they're given in hospital• *Genotyping of Drug Targets: A Method to Predict Adverse Drug Reactions?*, C Guzey, O Spigset, Drug Safety (25) 8, 2002

293 *phenylketonuria*• *NHS Choices*, NHS, URL-157, accessed December 7th 2011

293 improve hugely when they're given stimulants• *Catechol O-methyltransferase val158-met genotype and individual variation in the brain response to amphetamine*, Mattay et al, Proceedings of the National Academy of Sciences USA, 2003

294 Val-vals are less pain sensitive• *COMT val158met Genotype Affects u-Opioid Neurotransmitter Responses to a Pain Stressor*, Jon-Kar Zubieta et al, Science, February 2003

294 "warrior" type who is more willing to take risks, while met-mets are the "worriers", who are naturally more cautious• *Warriors versus worriers: the role of COMT gene variants*, DJ Stein, TK Newman, J Savitz, R Ramesar, CNS Spectrums, October 2006

295 between the publicly-funded Human Genome Project and the private company Celera Genomics• *The Human Genome Project*, The Wellcome Trust Sanger Institute, URL-158, accessed December 10th 2011

295 *Moore v Regents of the University of California*,• (271 Cal. Rptr.146), 1990

297 vaccines to make drugs ineffective• *Drugs and the Future: Brain Science, Addiction and Society*, David Nutt et al, Elsevier, 2007

298 Figure 16.2 compares treatment with D-cycloserine against treatment with a placebo• *Use of D-Cycloserine in Phobic Individuals to Facilitate Extinction of Fear*, Kerry J Ressler et al, Archives of General Psychiatry, 2004

299 alcohol craving can be reduced by using substance P antagonists• *Neurokinen 1 receptor antagonism as a possible therapy for alcoholism*, David George et al, Science, March 14th 2008

300 Alpha-5 receptors make you lose your memory• *Blockade of alcohol's amnestic activity in humans by an a5 subtype benzodiazepine receptor inverse agonist*, David Nutt et al, Neuropharmacology, 2007

300 inverse agonist•an inverse agonist is an agent that binds to the same receptor as a drug but induces a pharmacological response opposite to the drug. (Wikipedia.)

301 *Drugs and the Future*,• *Drugs and the Future: Brain Science, Addiction and Society*, David Nutt et al, Elsevier, 2007

17 What should I tell my kids about drugs?

All parents worry about their children trying drugs. I have four children myself, and know first-hand how difficult it is to balance keeping them safe and allowing them to start making decisions for themselves as they grow up. I first raised the topic with my eldest son when he was about thirteen, by which time he already knew a lot about drugs just from watching films and TV. With hindsight, I wish I'd started earlier, because he already had misconceptions about the benefits and risks. It's much easier to counter these if the conversations have been going on since childhood.

In many ways, it was probably easier for me than for most parents. The fact that I work with drugs meant that my children knew that I was well informed, and they trusted that I was telling them the truth. Of course, it's difficult to know if these conversations made a difference to their behaviour, because it's not a scientific experiment – you can't have a control case where you leave one child without any guidance at all! Hopefully, the information I gave them supported their own views that heroin and crack were very dangerous, and as a result none of them have ever experimented with them. While discussing drugs frankly with your children might not stop them experimenting with drugs, at least they will better understand what they are doing - and they know they can always come to you if they have a problem.

Young people and drugs

One of the most promising outcomes of the experiment with decriminalisation in Portugal has been a reduction in use of drugs by 15 to

19-year-olds. It is particularly risky for people to take drugs when they're young, as we'll explain in a moment. One important harm reduction measure is to *delay* experimentation, if it can't be prevented altogether. There are several reasons to try and discourage teenagers in particular from using drugs.

The first time you take any drug it will have a bigger effect on you, as you haven't developed any tolerance. For a young person who's relatively inexperienced about the world, this initial effect may be even more powerful, laying down the sorts of profoundly positive memories that can lead to addiction. It's also in adolescence that we lay the foundations for a lot of our habits, and teenage drug or alcohol use is a strong predictor for use in adulthood.

In general, young people are risk takers, and often appear to think they're immortal. Warning them about the dangers of dying a long time in the future – for example, from lung cancer if they start smoking now – doesn't act as much of a deterrent. Public-health campaigns targeting teenagers have now started focusing on the immediate downsides of habits (eg impotence or bad teeth from smoking) and this seems to be more effective than trying to get them to think about the long-term risks. Adolescents are also more likely than older people to do risky things when they're under the influence, which can put parents in a difficult position; as much as we want to discourage them from harmful activities, we also don't want them to try them secretly out on the street where they're much more likely to get into trouble.

Every child is different, and there's no single way to approach the issue, but below are 11 starting points for talking to your children about drugs.

1. Alcohol and tobacco are drugs

Most parents' number one fear is that their children will end up addicted to heroin or crack, and they start the conversation by explaining the dangers of "hard" drugs. In the process, children can often get the impression that alcohol and tobacco aren't really drugs, and aren't dangerous, when in many ways they're even more harmful than a lot of illegal substances, and smoking is highly addictive. Remember that [†]half of all regular smokers and a very large number of regular drinkers will die from illness caused by their alcohol or tobacco use, and with alcohol you don't have to be an addict to face considerable risks.

There's [†]no "safe level" of drinking and smoking, although some people drink and smoke in safer ways than others. Most of us have tried these drugs, and many of us use them regularly, weighing up the harms against the benefits we think we gain from them. Part of making adult decisions about drugs is learning how to weigh things up like this, and this is what we need to teach our children to do.

2. All drugs can potentially cause harm as well as pleasure

When you try a new drug, you can never be sure what its effects will be. There's often a chance you'll have a kind of "allergic reaction" and cause yourself real damage from a single experience. But even if you've taken something many times before, for all drugs the set and setting are so important that you can never entirely predict how you're going to react. If you're getting drugs on the street, there's the added danger of not knowing how strong something is or what it's been cut with. Even the drugs at the very bottom of the harms scale are never entirely safe; the best thing you can do to protect yourself is to make sure you're fully informed about what the risks are and have taken steps to minimise them.

3. Start telling your kids about drugs from an early age, and be prepared to discuss your drinking and smoking with them

Ideally, conversations about drugs should start when your children are six or seven – as they first become aware of drugs being used and discussed on TV and in films. Be prepared for them to already have a lot of ideas, both true and false, about how drugs work and what they do.

Make yourself a reliable source of information, so they'll come to you when they have questions. Part of making yourself reliable is being willing to discuss your own drug use – if you pretend that drinking and smoking are entirely different to the illegal substances they might be considering, they'll work out soon enough that this isn't true and you'll lose your credibility. Explain how you weigh up the risks and benefits when you're thinking about how much to drink or smoke, and under what circumstances you think certain kinds of use are appropriate.

4. Never inject

Injecting is by far the most risky route of use and you should *always* avoid it. Injecting drug users are at very high risk of infections and blood-borne viruses like HIV and hepatitis C, which are lifelong illnesses that will almost certainly do much more damage than the drug itself. Most drugs can be taken in some other way, and if someone really wants to experiment with a drug it's always better to use another method of getting it into the body instead of injecting it.

5. Don't use solvents

†Inhaling solvents, glue, butane or other aerosols kills about one person a week. They usually kill instantly, by stopping the heart, and this can happen the very first time the drug is tried. Solvents are popular amongst young teenagers because it's the easiest sort of substance to get hold of, but they're very dangerous to experiment with, even just once or twice. Make sure your kids know the harm they can do. (See box *Butane and other solvents* on page 315.)

6. Don't take drink and drugs at the same time

Mixing alcohol with other drugs makes the effects of both of them more unpredictable. There are two reasons for this, one chemical and the other social:

- Chemically, alcohol sometimes creates new compounds when combined with other drugs, such as cocaethylene which is produced when alcohol is mixed with cocaine. [†]Cocaethylene is more harmful than either drug on its own.

  Taking other kinds of depressants or opioids at the same time as alcohol is also dangerous as they can depress breathing to the point of death. You should be especially careful to avoid taking ketamine, GHB/GBL, heroin, methadone or any other opiate when you're drunk.

- The social element is that being drunk diminishes your judgement and makes you less careful about the other things you are taking. You may take the wrong drug (like the Scunthorpe Two, who wanted to try mephedrone but took methadone instead); you may also take a much higher dose than you would if you were sober. Warn your children to keep alcohol and other substances separate.

7. A criminal record could ruin your career

Even if you don't agree with the drug laws, you're still subject to them, and being caught in possession of drugs can get you into a lot of trouble. Sometimes the police might just confiscate or ignore small quantities of drugs, especially cannabis, but it's still a lottery. Some police still prosecute everyone they catch, and hundreds of thousands of people a year end up with a criminal record or even go to jail. Having a criminal record when you're young can badly affect your life. Just because you've got away with carrying drugs around many times before doesn't mean you won't be caught and prosecuted next time.

If you deal drugs, you're more likely to be targeted by the police and pursued through the courts, and the penalties are much more severe. Even passing on small amounts to your friends is considered dealing in the eyes of the law, so be extremely careful about doing that. Watch what you say and admit to online, as this could be used as evidence against you. Never post pictures of yourself or your friends doing illegal drugs.

8. Find good sources of advice

Unfortunately, there's an awful lot of misinformation about drugs, both on the internet and in the media. Any source that says "all drugs are evil" or "taking drugs is totally fine" is definitely not to be trusted! The scientific community does try to keep people informed, but this can be difficult as our knowledge is constantly changing and there are still so many unknowns. Our understanding of drugs and the brain is improving all the time, but there's still a lot we don't know about how drugs affect people on an individual level, and new designer drugs will inevitably keep hitting our streets. We've seen with mephedrone how the media can create scares that blow the harms of a new drug completely out of proportion. Perversely, this kind of scare-mongering can popularise new legal highs and make young people even more sceptical about the information they read in the papers. The danger is that when your kids discover how much the mainstream media exaggerate certain sort of harm they will turn to even less-reliable sources online.

We're trying to counteract this on the ISCD website, drugscience.org.uk, which has a lot of useful information written in an accessible style that teenagers should be able to understand without difficulty. We will keep this up-to-date as new substances appear. If you've found this book informative, do encourage them to read it too.

9. If you do take drugs (including alcohol and tobacco) be clear why you're doing it

There are lots of personal reasons people might want to take drugs – sometimes it's purely for pleasure, but often it's to deal with stress and anxiety. A great many people use alcohol in this way, when it would be far better to go to their GP and see if they can suggest a therapeutic drug or psychological approach which is less harmful and less addictive. Having a particularly strong liking for certain drugs can be an early indicator of mental-health problems – liking alcohol may be a sign of an anxiety problem, or liking cannabis may be an early indicator of

Drugs – without the hot air, David Nutt

schizophrenia. About [†]a quarter of male alcoholics have an undiagnosed anxiety disorder, and could have avoided damaging their bodies if they had been placed on a benzodiazepine or SSRI rather than self-medicating with what was available in the shops. If you do have a mental-health problem that you are dealing with by taking alcohol or illicit substances, you will do yourself much less harm if you move on to less addictive, medically-approved drugs under the guidance of a doctor or psychiatrist. If you think your child might be doing this, do try to get them a referral as soon as possible.

There are also social reasons for taking drugs, and there can be a lot of peer pressure to experiment when everyone else is doing it. This isn't limited to young people – adults can be very pushy about buying each other drinks in the pub – but teenagers are particularly sensitive to the approval of their peers and need to be supported in making their own decisions. Remind them that they are taking a risk with their own body every time they take drugs, and no one else should make that decision for them. Help them to resist peer pressure by encouraging them to read up on drugs so that they know about the risks they're exposing themselves to, rather than just relying on information from their friends who may be unaware what they're doing to themselves.

10. If you do get into trouble with drugs, get help quickly

If you do find yourself becoming physically or psychologically dependent on a drug, the longer you continue using it, the harder it will be for your brain to repair itself when you stop. The sooner you get help, the easier it will be to cope with your addiction. Your dependence is also likely to make you behave differently and make things difficult for your friends and family, just when you'll need their support most in battling the disease. Getting treatment before these relationships break down altogether will ensure that the treatment is much more likely to work.

If you think your child is developing a drug problem it can be extremely distressing, and very hard to know what to do. It might be tempting to try to force them into treatment, but the nature of addiction means that forcible interventions usually won't work: unless they're really motivated to come off the drugs themselves they're likely to relapse very quickly. There are no straightforward answers to this, but here are some suggestions:

- In the first instance discuss with your child your evidence and fears; educate them (perhaps with the material in this book) about the risks and harms of drugs.
- Then ask them what approach they would prefer (because without their agreement it can be hard to effect change). This could include discussion with friends who are using/supplying, teachers, GPs and church or other community figures that they respect and who have experience.
- Many GP practices have counsellors that may be able to help, or if not, who can direct you to local agencies that can. A search of the web will identify a huge number of treatment agencies for alcohol and drug users. While it can be hard to work out how all these agencies compare, a good place to start is the National Treatment Agency website, www.nta.nhs.uk
- Parental sanctions such as "grounding" or withdrawal of pocket money may be effective.
- Some parents choose to scare their children out of drug use by reporting them to the police. This is a high-risk strategy: the police may have to prosecute, which can result in a criminal record that can be more damaging to your child's prospects than the use of the drug, and can permanently damage their trust and respect in you.

11. If you do use drugs, make sure they don't interfere with your schoolwork

Experimenting with drugs can be really exciting, and may be more fun than going to school! If you're going to use drugs, it's really important to keep these parts of your life separate. Make sure the amount of time you spend doing drugs doesn't prevent you doing your homework, and that you're in a fit state to listen and pay attention in class – don't go in regularly with a hangover or keep missing sleep on school nights. Don't take drugs into school, or use them there, or deal on the school grounds: remember that just passing small amounts onto your friends will be seen as dealing. Even possessing legal drugs like alcohol will be against your school code of conduct, and could get you suspended or expelled.

School might seem like a waste of time now, but you can seriously damage your choices for the future if you fall behind in your work and waste your opportunities. Getting behind or getting yourself into trouble at school will probably be the biggest effect drugs have on your life.

Butane and other solvents

We've included information about solvents in this chapter because they are used mostly by young people, and are often the first intoxicating substance that young people try.

†Solvents are quite commonly abused by adolescents, because they're the easiest sort of drug to get hold of by young teenagers who can't yet buy alcohol legally. The solvents are either liquids or gases, which can be taken in a number of ways. Sometimes they are "huffed", which means placing some of the substance on a towel or cloth and breathing in; sometimes they are inhaled directly from the container; a third method is "bagging" – squirting the substance into a paper or plastic bag and inhaling. Aerosols are sometimes sprayed directly into the nose or mouth which is especially dangerous. How long the effect lasts depends on the substance – with some it lasts only a few minutes, and with others over an hour. The effects are quite like sudden drunkenness, with impaired coordination, lethargy and slurred speech, combined with light-headedness and euphoria.

Although butane, the solvent the ISCD expert panel looked at across the 16 criteria of harm, didn't score very highly overall, it's very unsafe to experiment with this type of drug. Solvent users can asphyxiate if they pass out while sedated and choke on their own vomit, or if they don't remove the cloth or bag from their face and continue to inhale the drug while they're unconscious. Long-term use can also cause brain damage, harm the liver and kidneys, and lead to hearing loss and convulsions or limb spasms. But the main danger is *sudden sniffing death syndrome* (SSDS), when a single session results in irregular heartbeat, heart failure and death. Over half of all deaths from solvents are from SSDS, and a fifth of those who died had no history of abusing inhalants. This makes it an extremely dangerous sort of drug to experiment with, even once or twice.

Many common household items like paint, glue and aerosols will give a kind of hit if they're inhaled. The only restriction on their sale is that shopkeepers aren't allowed to sell them to people they suspect might be intending to abuse them. It's very difficult to stop young people having access to them; the best thing we can do to protect children is explain the dangers and hope they make sensible decisions which will keep them safe.

Notes

Page

309 half of all regular smokers• *Mortality in relation to smoking: 50 years' observations on male British doctors*, Richard Doll et al, British Medical Journal (Clinical research ed.) 328, 2004

309 no "safe level" of drinking• *There is no such thing as a safe level of alcohol consumption*, David Nutt, URL-36, March 7th 2011

310 Inhaling solvents, glue, butane or other aerosols kills about one person a week.• *Trends in UK deaths associated with abuse of volatile substances*, Hamid Ghodse et al, International Centre for Drug Policy, 2010

311 Cocaethylene is more harmful than either drug on its own• *The Cocaine Trade*, House of Commons Home Affairs Committee, URL-110, February 23rd 2010

313 a quarter of male alcoholics have an undiagnosed anxiety disorder• *Comorbidity of Mental Disorders With Alcohol and Other Drug Abuse*, Darrel Regier et al, Journal of the American Medical Association (264), 1990

315 Solvents are quite commonly abused by adolescents,• *Legally Stoned*, Todd A Thies, Kensington Publishing Corp, 2009

URLs

Useful websites

- The *Independent Scientific Committee on Drugs* UK (ISCD):
  www.drugscience.org.uk
- The *Advisory Council on the Misuse of Drugs* UK:
  www.homeoffice.gov.uk/drugs/acmd
- The *National Institute on Drug Abuse* USA (NIDA):
  www.drugabuse.gov
- The *National Institute on Alcohol Abuse and Alcoholism* USA (NIAAA):
  www.niaaa.nih.gov
- The *National Drugs Campaign* Australia:
  www.drugs.health.gov.au

URLs referenced in the text

1. www.theyworkforyou.com/debate/?id=2011-07-13b.337.0
2. www.crimeandjustice.org.uk/opus1714/Estimating_drug_harms.pdf
3. www.drugscope.org.uk/Resources/Drugscope/Documents/PDF/virtuallibrary/
   runcimanreport.pdf
4. www.guardian.co.uk/politics/2009/nov/02/drug-policy-alan-johnson-nutt
5. www.timesonline.co.uk/tol/comment/columnists/guest_contributors/
   article6898671.ece
6. www.timesonline.co.uk/tol/life_and_style/health/article5916887.ece
7. www.bbc.co.uk/news/health-10990921
8. www.homeoffice.gov.uk/publications/alcohol-drugs/drugs/acmd1/mdma-report

9. www.newscientist.com/article/mg20126953.300-editorial-drugs-drive-politicians-out-of-their-minds.html

10. www.legislation.gov.uk/ukpga/1994/33/part/V/crossheading/powers-in-relation-to-raves

11. www.youtube.com/watch?v=a1PtQ67urG4

12. www.globalcommissionondrugs.org/Arquivos/Global_Com_Mike_Trace.pdf

13. en.wikisource.org/wiki/RAVE_Act

14. www.drugpolicy.org/news/2002/07/innocent-club-owners-young-people-vulnerable-under-rapidly-moving-rave-bill

15. www.horsedeathwatch.com/

16. www.thelancet.com/journals/lancet/article/PIIS0140-6736%2810%2961462-6/abstract

17. www.homeoffice.gov.uk/publications/alcohol-drugs/drugs/acmd1/ACMD-multi-criteria-report?view=Binary

18. www.catalyze.co.uk/?id=215

19. www.dailymail.co.uk/debate/article-1325788/Why-doesnt-Prof-David-Nutt-come-clean-admit-wants-legalise-drugs.html

20. www.bbc.co.uk/news/uk-11660210

21. www.homeoffice.gov.uk/publications/alcohol-drugs/drugs/acmd1/ ketamine-report.pdf?view=Binary

22. www.unodc.org/pdf/convention_1961_en.pdf

23. www.accionandina.org/documentos/Wonders-of-the-Coca-Leaf.pdf

24. www.who.int/bulletin/volumes/89/3/10-079905.pdf

25. www.nps.gov/history/local-law/fhpl_indianrelfreact.pdf

26. www.publications.parliament.uk/pa/ld199798/ldselect/ldsctech/151/15101.htm

27. www.beckleyfoundation.org/science/projects14.html

28. www.ukcia.org/culture/history/colonial.php

29. digital.nls.uk/indiapapers/browse/pageturner.cfm?id=74908458

30. profdavidnutt.wordpress.com/2010/12/13/necessity-or-nastiness-the-hidden-law-denying-cannabis-for-medicinal-use/

31. en.wikipedia.org/wiki/Barack_Obama

32. en.wikipedia.org/wiki/Use_of_performance-enhancing_drugs_in_sport

33. vimeo.com/23580287

34. www.ers.usda.gov/Publications/AGES001e/

35. www.alcoholconcern.org.uk/assets/files/Publications/
    Swept%20under%20the%20carpet.pdf
36. www.guardian.co.uk/science/2011/mar/07/safe-level-alcohol-consumption
37. m.guardian.co.uk/commentisfree/2010/nov/05/alcohol-drug-worse-than-heroin?
    cat=commentisfree&type=article
38. www.ic.nhs.uk/webfiles/publications/alcohol10/Statistics_on_Alcohol_England_
    2010.pdf
39. www.eucam.info/eucam/home/marketing-products-and-reports.html?
    bericht2248=1099
40. www.bma.org.uk/health_promotion_ethics/alcohol/undertheinfluence.jsp
41. www.cedro-uva.org/lib/levine.alcohol.html
42. www.policyexchange.org.uk/images/publications/pdfs/
    Cough_Up_-_March__10.pdf
43. www.guardian.co.uk/politics/2011/may/28/
    andrew-lansley-u-turn-public-health-cuts
44. profdavidnutt.wordpress.com/2011/01/19/teaching-the-tricks-of-the-liquor-trade/
45. m.guardian.co.uk/education/2009/nov/08/philip-laing-carnage-binge-drinking?
    cat=education&type=article
46. www.ias.org.uk/resources/factsheets/drink_driving.pdf
47. www.reuters.com/article/2008/07/01/
    us-minimum-drinking-age-idUSARM15193120080701
48. www.bbc.co.uk/news/10184803
49. www.telegraph.co.uk/news/uknews/7521446/Teenagers-death-latest-linked-
    to-mephedrone.html
50. news.sky.com/home/uk-news/article/15501782
51. www.thesun.co.uk/sol/homepage/news/2747979/
    Lad-ripped-his-scrotum-off.html
52. m.guardian.co.uk/media/2010/apr/05/
    mephedrone-drug-media-scare-newspapers?cat=media&type=article
53. www.drugscience.org.uk/mephedronescience.html
54. www.eveningtelegraph.co.uk/output/2010/05/31/story15149404t0.shtm
55. www.injuryobservatory.net/documents/npSAD10thdeathreport.pdf
56. www.straightstatistics.org/article/
    banned-drug-may-have-saved-lives-not-cost-them

57. www.straightstatistics.org/article/mephedrone-and-cocaine-clues-army-testing

58. blogs.telegraph.co.uk/news/christopherhope/100033336/ban-on-miaow-miaow-party-drug-could-cost-britain-600million-in-lost-import-duty/

59. ndarc.med.unsw.edu.au/sites/all/shared_files/ndarc/resources/EDRS%20Bulletin%20Dec%202010.pdf

60. www.thelancet.com/journals/lancet/article/PIIS0140-6736(10)60556-9/fulltext

61. news.bbc.co.uk/1/hi/uk/8601315.stm

62. www.thisisscunthorpe.co.uk/Decision-outlaw-drug-connected-deaths/story-11171980-detail/story.html

63. www.thelancet.com/journals/lancet/article/PIIS0140-6736(10)62021-1/fulltext

64. www.newscientist.com/mobile/article/dn18712-miaowmiaow-on-trial-truth-or-trumpedup-charges.html

65. www.bbc.co.uk/newsbeat/10353130

66. transform-drugs.blogspot.com/2010/03/mephedrone-and-acmd-lessons-from-bzp.html?m=1

67. www.homeoffice.gov.uk/publications/alcohol-drugs/drugs/temporary-bans/temporary-class-drugs?view=Binary

68. m.guardian.co.uk/commentisfree/2010/mar/17/mephedrone-class-d-solution-criminalise?cat=commentisfree&type=article

69. www.drugscience.org.uk/minimumdataset.html

70. www.emcdda.europa.eu/html.cfm/index132196EN.html

71. profdavidnutt.wordpress.com/2010/05/28/scunthorpe-two/

72. www.homeoffice.gov.uk/publications/alcohol-drugs/drugs/acmd1/khat-report-2005/Khat_Report_.pdf?view=Binary

73. www.camh.net/education/Resources_communities_organizations/stigma_subabuse_litreview99.pdf

74. www.guardian.co.uk/music/2011/may/20/pete-doherty-jailed-six-months

75. www.people.com/people/article/0,,20243428,00.html

76. www.telegraph.co.uk/news/celebritynews/1937076/Amy-Winehouse-bailed-over-drugs-video.html

77. content.usatoday.com/communities/entertainment/post/2011/09/amy-winehouse-died-after-detox-seizure-dad-says/1

78. www.who.int/substance_abuse/publications/en/PositionPaper_English.pdf

79. www.guardian.co.uk/society/2010/apr/20/

conservatives-heroin-addiction-treatment-overhaul

80. profdavidnutt.wordpress.com/2010/06/09/
crutch-or-cure-the-realities-of-methadone-treatment/

81. www.cato.org/pubs/wtpapers/greenwald_whitepaper.pdf

82. www.guardian.co.uk/world/2010/sep/05/portugal-drugs-debate

83. www.soros.org/initiatives/drugpolicy/articles_publications/publications/
drug-policy-in-portugal-20110829/drug-policy-in-portugal-20110829.pdf

84. www.telegraph.co.uk/culture/qi/6833236/QI-quite-interesting-facts-about-wine.
html

85. en.wikipedia.org/wiki/Crack_cocaine#Chemistry

86. m.guardian.co.uk/world/2008/nov/19/
cocaine-rainforests-columbia-santos-calderon?cat=world&type=article

87. www.bbc.co.uk/news/world-latin-america-12177875

88. collections.europarchive.org/tna/20110202220654/http://www.smokefreeengland.
co.uk/what-do-i-do/quick-guide.html

89. www.independent.co.uk/life-style/health-and-families/health-news/smoking-ban-
has-saved-40000-lives-856885.html

90. www.who.int/mediacentre/factsheets/fs339/en/index.html

91. www.who.int/tobacco/statistics/tobacco_atlas/en/

92. news.bbc.co.uk/onthisday/hi/dates/stories/november/18/
newsid_2519000/2519675.stm

93. www.advisorybodies.doh.gov.uk/scoth/PDFs/scothnov2004.pdf

94. www.surgeongeneral.gov/library/secondhandsmoke/report/fullreport.pdf

95. www.gutenberg.org/files/17008/17008-h/17008-h.htm

96. www.youtube.com/watch?v=gCMzjJjuxQI

97. legacy.library.ucsf.edu/tid/qxp91e00/pdf

98. www.ons.gov.uk/ons/rel/mro/news-release/
seventy-years-of-social-surveys/socsurv02092011-nr.html

99. www.publications.parliament.uk/pa/cm200506/cmselect/cmhealth/485/48506.
htm

100. www.ons.gov.uk/ons/rel/cancer-unit/cancer-incidence-and-mortality/2006-2008/
index.html

101. www.cancer.org/Cancer/CancerCauses/TobaccoCancer/WomenandSmoking/
women-and-smoking-intro

102. www.nhs.uk/news/2010/06June/Pages/Heart-attacks-fall-after-smoking-ban. aspx

103. Opposingthe-UK-smokingban.org

104. www.reuters.com/article/2009/07/31/ us-smoking-odd-idUSTRE56U4BO20090731

105. www.badscience.net/2011/03/why-cigarette-packs-matter/

106. cgch.lshtm.ac.uk/tobacco/Handbook%2008.07.03.pdf

107. info.cancerresearchuk.org/healthyliving/smokingandtobacco/passivesmoking/

108. www.homeoffice.gov.uk/publications/science-research-statistics/ research-statistics/crime-research/hosb1211/hosb1211?view=Binary

109. www.ic.nhs.uk/webfiles/publications/003_Health_Lifestyles/Statistics%20on% 20Smoking%202011/Statistics_on_Smoking_2011.pdf

110. www.publications.parliament.uk/pa/cm200910/cmselect/cmhaff/74/74i.pdf

111. webarchive.nationalarchives.gov.uk/20110218135832/http://rds.homeoffice.gov. uk/rds/pdfs06/rdsolr1606.pdf

112. www.who.int/tobacco/en/atlas16.pdf

113. www.dailymail.co.uk/health/article-2042963/Tens-1000s-surgical-patients-die-needlessly-poor-NHS-care.html?ITO=1490

114. www.guardian.co.uk/sport/2009/jul/26/tour-de-france-tom-simpson-tributes

115. www.homeoffice.gov.uk/publications/alcohol-drugs/drugs/acmd1/ anabolic-steroids-report/anabolic-steroids?view=Binary

116. www.nytimes.com/2003/09/10/sports/sprinter-likely-to-lose-medals.html

117. www.telegraph.co.uk/sport/4532637/ Michael-Phelps-suspended-for-three-months-over-bong-photograph.html

118. www.nimh.nih.gov/health/publications/schizophrenia/complete-index.shtml

119. www.telegraph.co.uk/travel/destinations/europe/turkey/8678795/Wake-up-and-smell-the-coffee-in-Turkeys-beautiful-Izmir.html

120. www.youtube.com/watch?v=UQP1IsAv1jg

121. thephoenix.com/boston/news/62230-will-harvard-drop-acid-again/

122. www.time.com/time/magazine/article/0,9171,905238,00.html

123. www.bbc.co.uk/blogs/thereporters/markeaston/2010/12/can_we_imagine_a_ britain_where.html

124. www.tdpf.org.uk/strategy_unit_drugs_report.pdf

125. www.globalcommissionondrugs.org/Report

126. www.tdpf.org.uk/strategy_unit_drugs_report.pdf
127. www.justice.gov.uk/downloads/publications/statistics-and-data/mojstats/2011-compendium-reoffending-stats-analysis.pdf
128. dassa.sa.gov.au/webdata/resources/files/monograph6.pdf
129. www.gao.gov/new.items/d03172r.pdf
130. www.surgeongeneral.gov/library/youthviolence/chapter5/sec4.html
131. www.tdpf.org.uk/Transform_After_the_War_on_Drugs.pdf
132. www.tdpf.org.uk/Policy_General_Strategy_Unit_Drugs_Report_phase_1.htm
133. www.unaids.org/en/strategygoalsby2015/injectingdruguseandhiv/
134. www.nytimes.com/2011/01/17/world/europe/17russia.html?_r=1&partner=rss&emc=rss
135. blog.soros.org/2011/01/russias-hiv-care-must-center-on-drug-users/
136. www.youtube.com/watch?v=kCtxrm4cWPM
137. www.internationalreporting.org/blog/2011/07/07/the-pain-project/
138. m.guardian.co.uk/world/2011/apr/03/us-bank-mexico-drug-gangs?cat=world&type=article
139. www.bbc.co.uk/news/world-latin-america-10681249
140. www.huffingtonpost.com/2008/10/16/al-qaedas-drug-trade-keep_n_135352.html
141. www.cbc.ca/news/world/story/2011/08/28/f-mexico-drug-cartels.html
142. www.unodc.org/unodc/en/frontpage/assisting-guinea-bissau.html
143. www.publications.parliament.uk/pa/cm200910/cmselect/cmpubacc/456/456.pdf
144. www.ncbi.nlm.nih.gov/pmc/articles/PMC1846683/pdf/brmedj02604-0038.pdf
145. www.who.int/tobacco/health_priority/en/
146. www.who.int/substance_abuse/publications/global_alcohol_report/msbgsruprofiles.pdf
147. www.unodc.org/documents/data-and-analysis/WDR2011/Global_and_regional_overview.pdf
148. www.foxnews.com/world/2010/05/13/ap-impact-years-trillion-war-drugs-failed-meet-goals/
149. news.bbc.co.uk/1/hi/uk_politics/1955789.stm
150. www.independent.co.uk/news/uk/politics/tory-contender-calls-for-more-liberal-

drug-laws-505824.html

151. www.tdpf.org.uk/Policy_General_AftertheWaronDrugsReport.htm

152. www.mind.org.uk/help/rights_and_legislation/statistics_8_the_criminal_justice_system

153. www.dailymail.co.uk/news/article-1320494/Kenneth-Clarke-Return-Victorian-style-prisons-hard-work-NO-drugs.html

154. research.dwp.gov.uk/asd/asd5/rrep155.pdf

155. www.independent.co.uk/news/uk/crime/ken-clarke-plans-radical-reform-of-the-prison-system-2014307.html

156. www.child-soldiers.org

157. www.nhs.uk/conditions/Phenylketonuria/Pages/Introduction.aspx

158. www.sanger.ac.uk/about/history/hgp/

159. www.bbc.co.uk/news/uk-16342906

160. www.publications.parliament.uk/pa/cm200607/cmselect/cmsctech/uc65-i/uc6502.htm

161. www.drugs.homeoffice.gov.uk/publication-search/acmd/acmd-cannabis-report-2008

162. www.publications.parliament.uk/pa/cm200910/cmselect/cmhealth/151/151i.pdf

163. download.thelancet.com/pdfs/journals/lancet/PIIS0140673611605126.pdf

164. www.ecnp.eu/~/media/Files/ecnp/communication/reports/ECNP%20EBC%20Report.ashx

165. jop.sagepub.com/content/26/2/205.full.pdf+html

166. www.google.co.uk/trends/?q=mephedrone+deaths,+mephedrone+buy

167. www.homeoffice.gov.uk/acmd1/acmd-cathinodes-report-2010?view=Binary

168. www.guardian.co.uk/world/2010/mar/05/korean-girl-starved-online-game

169. www.drugabuse.gov/sites/default/files/sciofaddiction.pdf

170. info.cancerresearchuk.org/prod_consump/groups/cr_common/@nre/@sta/documents/generalcontent/crukmig_1000ast-2989.xls

171. www.pnas.org/cgi/doi/10.1073/pnas.1119598109

172. www.guardian.co.uk/society/2010/oct/31/race-bias-drug-arrests-claim

173. www.nytimes.com/2011/06/17/opinion/17carter.html

174. www.guardian.co.uk/politics/2007/feb/11/uk.drugsandalcohol1

175. www.ukcia.org/research/ProjectionsOfImpactOfRiseInUse/ProjectionsOfImpactOfRiseInUse.pdf

176. www.beckleyfoundation.org/2011/11/19/public-letter-in-the-times-and-guardian-calling-for-a-new-approach
177. www.homeoffice.gov.uk/drugs/drug-law/
178. www.time.com/time/world/article/0,8599,1887488,00.html
179. www.apa.org/science/programs/conference/2011/harwood.ppt
180. www.msnbc.msn.com/id/35914759/ns/business-world_business/t/wachovia-settle-drug-money-laundering-case
181. www.dailymail.co.uk/news/article-435393/Exclusive-Cameron-DID-smoke-cannabis.html
182. www.lawrencephillips.net/Decision_conferencing.html

Index

Page numbers in **bold** indicate definitions.

attention deficit hyperactivity disorder,
  see ADHD
auditory effects, schizophrenia, 254
Australia, decriminalisation of drugs in,
  272
ayuesca, psychedelic, 57

baby, starved by parents, 137
baclofen, 107
bagging, route of use, 315
ban, temporary order, 122
banisteriopsis caapi, **259**
banks, money-laundering, 276
barbiturates, 217, 218, 221
  PTSD, and, 264
  suicide, 217
Barcelona, 114
battle fatigue, 264, *see also* PTSD
BCS, *see* British Crime Survey
benefits
  cannabis, 74
  mephedrone, 117
  psychedelics, 255
Benzedrine, 265, 266
benzodiazepines, 38, 217–221
  addiction, 218
  alcohol treatment, in, 218
  benefits, 217–221
  depressant, 57
  endogenous, 217
  GABA receptors, 217
  harms, 217–221
  how they work, 217
  Librium, 217
  overdose, safer, 217
  physical dependence, 218
  rebound less likely, 223
  side effects, few, 218

suicide and, 218
withdrawal, 218
benzylpiperazine, 121
Bernays, Edward, 203
beta blockers in sport, 237
Betts, Leah, 15, 117
bhang, 74, 79
binge
  cocaine, 140
  drinking, 5, 95, 108
  LSD, impossible, 141
  tolerance and, 140
  treatment, 161
Bird, Sheila, Professor, 117
bladder, ketamine, 33
Blair, Tony, 281
blind trial, **226**
Bolivia, 181, 188
  coca, 66, 187
bong, 77
brain
  addiction mechanisms, 135
  default mode, 248
brain chemicals, 51
  receptors, 134
Brain Science, Addiction and Drugs
      programme, 300–305
    dispense with care scenario, 303
    high performance scenario, 301
    neighbourhood watch scenario, 302
    treated positively scenario, 304
Brake, Tom, MP, 1
Breakdown Britain, 167, 173
British Aerobatic Association, 237
British Crime Survey, 234
Brokenshire, James, 84
bromides, PTSD, and, 264

Drugs – without the hot air, David Nutt

Drugs – without the hot air, David Nutt

Drugs – without the hot air, David Nutt

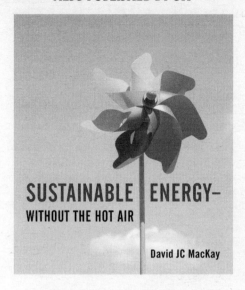

SUSTAINABLE ENERGY–
WITHOUT THE HOT AIR

David JC MacKay

ISBN (paperback) 9780954452933
ISBN (hardback) 9781906860011
384 pages, full colour throughout

"This book is a tour de force ... as a work of popular science it is exemplary"
The Economist

"This is to energy and climate what Freakonomics is to economics."
Cory Doctorow, boingboing.net

"This year's must-read book about tackling our future energy needs."
The Guardian

"If someone wants an overall view of how energy gets used, where it comes from, and the challenges in switching to new sources, this is the book to read. ... I was thrilled to see a book that is scientific, numeric, broad, open-minded, and well written on a topic where a lot of narrow, obscure, non-numeric writing confuses the public. People need to really understand what is going on and then be part of the process of moving the world to a new energy infrastructure."
Bill Gates

ALSO PUBLISHED BY UIT

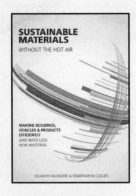

ISBN, 9781906860301
416 pages, paperback

"a pragmatic guide to getting more value from less stuff."
BBC News Magazine

"essential reading for both student and practitioner"
Materials World

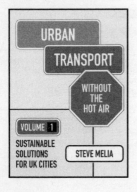

ISBN, 9781906860264
264 pages, paperback

"A fresh perspective on urban transport"
Sir Peter Hendy, Chairman of Network Rail, former Commissioner of Transport for London

ALSO PUBLISHED BY UIT

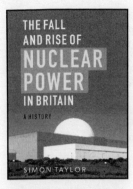

ISBN, 9781906860318
256 pages, paperback

"a terrific piece of work... far greater and more devastating in detail than anything else so far in the public domain"
Lord Howell, former Secretary of State for Energy

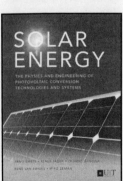

ISBN, 9781906860325
488 pages, paperback

The book is an excellent companion to the Massive Open Online Course (MOOC) on Solar Energy (by one the book's authors), which has won the OpenCourseWare Excellence Award 2014. An invaluable reference for researchers, industrial engineers and designers working in Solar Energy

Join our mailing list

Information every month or two, about new books,
author appearances, events, podcasts, and
topics of interest. To join:

www.uit.co.uk/subscribe

Tell us what you think

To contact us about any of our books, or
if you're interesting in writing a book:

www.uit.co.uk/contact